Cardiology

Guest Editor

J. JILL HEATLEY, DVM, MS,
Dipl. ABVP–Avian, Dipl. ACZM

VETERINARY CLINICS OF NORTH AMERICA: EXOTIC ANIMAL PRACTICE

www.vetexotic.theclinics.com

Consulting Editor
AGNES E. RUPLEY, DVM, Dipl. ABVP–Avian

January 2009 • Volume 12 • Number 1

SAUNDERS an imprint of ELSEVIER, Inc.

W.B. SAUNDERS COMPANY

A Division of Elsevier Inc.

1600 John F. Kennedy Boulevard ● Suite 1800 ● Philadelphia, Pennsylvania 19103-2899

http://www.vetexotic.theclinics.com

**VETERINARY CLINICS OF NORTH AMERICA: EXOTIC ANIMAL PRACTICE Volume 12, Number 1
January 2009 ISSN 1094-9194, ISBN-13: 978-1-4377-0557-7, ISBN-10: 1-4377-0557-X**

Editor: John Vassallo; j.vassallo@elsevier.com

Veterinary Clinics of North America: Exotic Animal Practice (ISSN 1094-9194) is published in January, May, and September by Elsevier, Inc.; Business and Editorial offices: 1600 John F. Kennedy Blvd., Suite 1800, Philadelphia, PA 19103-2899. Customer Service Office: 11830 Westline Industrial Drive, St. Louis, MO 63146. Subscription prices are $180.00 per year for US individuals, $323.00 per year for US institutions, $94.00 per year for US students and residents, $213.00 per year for Canadian individuals, $381.00 per year for Canadian institutions, $240.00 per year for international individuals, $381.00 per year for international institutions and $120.00 per year for Canadian and foreign students/residents. To receive student/resident rate, orders must be accompanied by name of affiliated institution, date of term, and the *signature* of program/residency coordinator on institution letterhead. Orders will be billed at individual rate until proof of status is received. Foreign air speed delivery is included in all *Clinics* subscription prices. All prices are subject to change without notice. **POSTMASTER:** Send address changes to *Veterinary Clinics of North America: Exotic Animal Practice*, 11830 Westline Industrial Drive, St. Louis, MO 63146. Customer Service (orders, claims, online, change of address): Elsevier Periodicals **Customer Service, 11830 Westline Industrial Drive, St. Louis, MO 63146. Tel: 1-800-654-2452 (U.S. and Canada); 314-453-7041 (outside U.S. and Canada). Fax: 314-523-5170. E-mail: journalscustomerservice-usa@elsevier. com (for print support); journalsonlinesupport-usa@elsevier (for online support).**

Reprints. For copies of 100 or more of articles in this publication, please contact the commercial Reprints Department, Elsevier Inc., 360 Park Avenue South, New York, New York 10010-1710. Tel: (212) 633-3813 Fax: (212) 633-1935, E-mail: reprints@elsevier.com.

Veterinary Clinics of North America: Exotic Animal Practice is covered in *MEDLINE/PubMed (Index Medicus)*.

Printed and bound by CPI Group (UK) Ltd, Croydon, CR0 4YY

Transferred to Digital Print 2011

Contributors

CONSULTING EDITOR

AGNES E. RUPLEY, DVM
Diplomate, American Board of Veterinary Practitioners–Avian Practice; and Director and Chief Veterinarian, All Pets Medical Center, College Station, Texas

GUEST EDITOR

J. JILL HEATLEY, DVM, MS
Diplomate, American Board of Veterinary Practitioners–Avian, Diplomate, American College of Zoological Medicine; Clinical Associate Professor, Department of Small Animal Clinical Sciences, Zoological Medicine Service, College of Veterinary Medicine, Texas A&M University, College Station, Texas

AUTHORS

J. JILL HEATLEY, DVM, MS
Diplomate, American Board of Veterinary Practitioners–Avian, Diplomate, American College of Zoological Medicine; Clinical Associate Professor, Department of Small Animal Clinical Sciences, Zoological Medicine Service, College of Veterinary Medicine, Texas A&M University, College Station, Texas

KATHLEEN M. HEINZ-TAHENY, DVM, PhD
Diplomate, American College of Veterinary Pathologists; Principal Research Pathologist, Lilly Research Laboratories, Eli Lilly and Co., Indianapolis, Indiana

STEPHEN HERNANDEZ-DIVERS, BVetMed, DZooMed
Member, Royal College of Veterinary Surgeons, Zoological Medicine; Department of Small Animal Medicine and Surgery, College of Veterinary Medicine, University of Georgia, Athens, Georgia

MARIA-ELISABETH KRAUTWALD-JUNGHANNS, DrMedVet
Diplomate, European College of Avian Medicine and Surgery; Professor and Director, Clinic for Birds and Reptiles, University of Leipzig, Leipzig, Germany

GARY D. MARTY, DVM, PhD
Diplomate, American College of Veterinary Pathologists; Research Associate, Department of Anatomy, Physiology, and Cell Biology, University of California, School of Veterinary Medicine, Davis, California; and Fish Pathologist, Ministry of Agriculture and Lands, Animal Health Centre, Abbotsford, British Columbia, Canada

MARK A. MITCHELL, DVM, MS, PhD
Associate Professor, Zoological Medicine, Department of Veterinary Clinical Medicine, University of Illinois, College of Veterinary Medicine, Urbana, Illinois

ROMAIN PARIAUT, DVM
Diplomate, American College of Veterinary Internal Medicine–Cardiology, European College of Veterinary Internal Medicine-Companion Animals–Cardiology; Assistant Professor of Cardiology, Department of Clinical Sciences, School of Veterinary Medicine, Louisiana State University, Baton Rouge, Louisiana

MICHAEL PEES, DrMedVet
Diplomate, European College of Avian Medicine and Surgery; Clinic for Birds and Reptiles, University of Leipzig, Leipzig, Germany

JOHANNA SHERRILL, DVM, MS
Diplomate, American College of Zoological Medicine; Companion and Exotic Animal Relief Veterinarian, Monterey, California

ROBERT A. WAGNER, VMD
Associate Professor of Veterinary Medicine; and Chief of Surgical Veterinary Services, Division of Laboratory Animal Resources, University of Pittsburgh, Pennsylvania

E. SCOTT WEBER III, VMD, MSc
Companion Avian and Exotic Animal Service, Department of Aquatic Animal Health, University of California, Medicine and Epidemiology, Davis, California

DAVID WILLIAMS, MA, VetMB, PhD, CertVOphthal, FRCVS
Associate Lecturer, Department of Veterinary Medicine, University of Cambridge; and Fellow and Director of Studies, Veterinary Medicine and Pathology, St John's College, Cambridge

JEANETTE WYNEKEN, PhD
Associate Professor, Department of Biological Sciences, Florida Atlantic University, Boca Raton, Florida

Contents

It may seem ridiculous to consider cardiac diseases in sub-vertebrate animals; when on earth is a tarantula, a butterfly or a snail going to be presented as a clinical case with heart failure or a congenital cardiac abnormality? This article examines the work of research groups investigating invertebrates as valuable models of heart disease in man. Examining invertebrates with gene defects similar to those in human patients with heart disease, congenital or acquired, allows us to probe deeply into the aetio-pathogenesis of many cardiac conditions.

Fish patients with cardiovascular disorders present a challenge in terms of diagnostic evaluation and therapeutic options. Veterinarians can approach these cases in fish using methods similar to those employed for other companion animals. Clinicians who evaluate and treat fish in private, aquarium, zoologic, or aquaculture settings need to rely on sound clinical judgment after thorough historical and physical evaluation. Pharmacokinetic data and treatments specific to cardiovascular disease in fish are limited; thus, drug types and dosages used in fish are largely empiric. Fish cardiovascular anatomy, physiology, diagnostic evaluation, monitoring, common diseases, cardiac pathologic conditions, formulary options, and comprehensive references are presented with the goal of providing fish veterinarians with clinically relevant tools.

The class Amphibia includes three orders of amphibians: the anurans (frogs and toads), urodeles (salamanders, axolotls, and newts), and caecilians. The diversity of lifestyles across these three orders has accompanying differences in the cardiovascular anatomy and physiology allowing for adaptations to aquatic or terrestrial habitats, pulmonic or gill respiration, hibernation, and body elongation (in the caecilian). This article provides a review of amphibian cardiovascular anatomy and physiology with discussion of unique species adaptations. In addition, amphibians as cardiovascular animal models and commonly encountered natural diseases are covered.

Major differences among reptile taxa include the shape of the heart, degree of separation of the ventricular compartments, degree of development of the intraventricular muscular ridge, and in crocodilians, the interventricular septum. In many cases, the structural-functional features of the reptilian heart provide adaptive plasticity, allowing for the ecological and behavioral diversity seen. As a result, variation may surface in clinical measures of cardiac performance. This article updates clinical context, provides an understanding of the variation in reptilian cardiovascular systems, and their functional implications for the assessment and treatment of reptile patients.

Cardiovascular disease in reptiles generally is considered an uncommon finding in captive animals, but no large-scale, cross-sectional studies have been performed to determine its prevalence. It is possible that cardiovascular disease is more common than is generally accepted and that the current belief results from limited clinical and diagnostic experience. This article offers guidance drawn from the author's clinical experience and the available literature. It is important that veterinarians pursue a thorough history, physical examination, and diagnostic work-up when managing cardiovascular disease in a reptile case. Veterinarians working with these cases should document their findings and share them with their colleagues to build an evidence-based foundation for reptile medicine.

Avian cardiac disease in pet birds occurs more often than previously assumed. The article focuses on anatomic peculiarities of the avian cardiovascular system and common diseases. Diagnostic possibilities are demonstrated, and therapeutic measures are discussed.

Cardiovascular disease in small exotic mammals is anecdotally common, but clinical reports of diagnosis and treatment of disease are rare. This article focuses on known causes of cardiovascular disease in the small exotic mammal. Normal anatomy and physiology, as it differs from the dog and cat, is also highlighted. Cardiomyopathy, dirofilariasis, atrial thrombosis, and other acquired and congenital cardiac and vascular diseases of rodents, hedgehogs, sugar gliders, raccoons, opossums, and skunks are reviewed. Expected clinical signs and diagnostic and treatment options, including a formulary, are provided for these species.

Cardiac disease in pet ferrets is common and includes dilated cardiomyopathy, arrhythmias, and acquired valvular disease. Clinical presentation of cardiac disease in ferrets may be similar to dog or cats, although hind limb weakness may be a prominent feature. Radiography, ECG, and ultrasound are all useful tools in the diagnosis of cardiac disease in ferrets. Therapeutics for cardiac disease in ferrets is based on recommendations for dogs and cats. The prognosis for cardiac disease in ferrets varies from fair to guarded, depending on underlying disease.

This article reviews what is known about the diagnosis and management of cardiovascular diseases in the pet rabbit. Current knowledge is based on anecdotal reports, derived from research data using the rabbit as an animal model of human cardiovascular diseases, but most importantly canine and feline cardiology. It is likely that, as cardiovascular diseases are more often recognized, more specific information will soon become available for the treatment of the pet rabbit with cardiac disease.

FORTHCOMING ISSUES

RECENT ISSUES

RELATED INTEREST

Veterinary Clinics of North America: Small Animal Practice (Volume 38, Issue 3, May 2008)
Advances in Fluid, Electrolyte, and Acid-Base Disorders
Helio Autran de Morais, DVM, PhD, and Stephen P. DiBartola, DVM, *Guest Editors*

THE CLINICS ARE NOW AVAILABLE ONLINE!

Access your subscription at:
www.theclinics.com

Preface

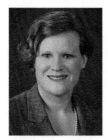

J. Jill Heatley, DVM, MS, DABVP–Avian, DACZM
Guest Editor

This issue of *Veterinary Clinics of North America: Exotic Animal Practice* focuses on cardiology of exotic animal species. While knowledge of cardiovascular disease in the cat and dog continues to advance rapidly, a number of factors hamper diagnosis and treatment of cardiovascular disease in the pet exotic animal. Cardiovascular physiology of these animals and normal values are seldom reviewed or are not easily available to the general practitioner. Thus, determining abnormal and subsequent diagnosis is hindered by the lack of knowledge of normal. Additionally, many of these animals lack clinical signs or have nondiscernable clinical signs based on their natural stoic defensive nature as prey species. Finally, the application of standard diagnostics may be made difficult by a lack of knowledge of basic physiology of this variety of creatures.

Articles included here are meant to present the leading edge of knowledge related to cardiovascular anatomy, physiology, diagnostics, and treatment in small exotic mammals, fish, reptiles, and invertebrates. While some of these articles lack clinical relevance at present, they represent what is known physiologically and provide a base for further expansion of knowledge.

Certainly cardiovascular disease is present in many exotic animals and is common based on pathology reviews. However, reports of detection antemortem and, even further, reports of treatment, are sadly lacking. This collection of reviews should serve not only as a signpost of current knowledge but also, and possibly more importantly, as a marker of what remains unknown in this field. I sincerely hope that this volume serves as impetus to many veterinarians to publish and share their successes and failures in dealing with cardiovascular diseases of exotic animals and will spur a sorely needed expansion of practical clinical knowledge in the field of exotic animal cardiovascular physiology, diagnosis, and treatment.

Finally, I should personally note that I am not a cardiologist, nor do I presume to have any special knowledge in this area. I began this journey based on a series of cases of ferret cardiac disease presented at the Auburn University College of Veterinary Medicine. These cases brought to my attention not only my clinical weakness in this area, but also the lack of clinical literature surrounding cardiovascular diseases in exotic animal species. I would like to personally thank Dr. Ray Dillon, whose clinical support with these initial cases, which included a willingness to apply the basic principles of cardiovascular treatment to ferrets, spurred my quest for continued knowledge, resulting in this work and other publications related to exotic animal cardiovascular disease.

J. Jill Heatley, DVM, MS, DABVP–Avian, DACZM
Diplomate American Board of Veterinary Practitioners–Avian
Diplomate American College of Zoological Medicine
Department of Veterinary Small Animal Clinical Sciences
College of Veterinary Medicine
Texas A&M University
4474-TAMU
College Station, TX 77843-4474, USA

E-mail address:
JHeatley@cvm.tamu.edu

Cardiac Biology and Disease in Invertebrates

David Williams, MA, VetMB, PhD, CertVOphthal, FRCVS[a,b,*]

KEYWORDS

• Cardiac • Invertebrate • Model • Genetic • Defect

It may seem ridiculous to consider cardiac diseases in sub-vertebrate animals; when on earth is a tarantula, a butterfly or a snail going to be presented as a clinical case with heart failure or a congenital cardiac abnormality? This review examines the work of research groups investigating invertebrates as valuable models of heart disease in man. "Ontogeny recapitulates phylogeny," or so the old adage goes. And nowhere is this truer than in the heart. We will review the evolution of the four-chambered heart from the primordial heart tube seen in primitive invertebrates and see how the development of the embryonic vertebrate heart parallels this evolutionary advancement.

THE INVERTEBRATE HEART—ANATOMY AND PHYSIOLOGY

The circulation in vertebrates, relatively large organisms compared to most invertebrates, transports oxygen, nutrients, and messenger molecules around the body. In the incredibly diverse world of invertebrates, the vascular system may indeed fulfill those roles, but also acts as a central part of supportive and locomotory structures in many species. It gives volume to snail's feet, opens the wings of butterflies emerging from their cocoons, and its pulsatile nature aids air movement in the tracheae of many arthropods. Most invertebrates have low oxygen requirements and little need for an advanced efficient pumping system for hemolymph distribution. Others, from flies to cephalopods, are rapid movers with high oxygen demand and highly evolved, efficient hearts. The problem is that the blood of these advanced invertebrates has a low oxygen carrying capacity. Cardiac output in these animals has to be very high to fuel the metabolic demands of such rapidly moving creatures as *Nautilus*. This particular species has a higher cardiac output than an active fish, such as the trout. The annelids, with their metabolic demands at the other end of the spectrum, can rely on their poorly contractile dorsal heart tube, the key primitive cardiac system,

a Department of Veterinary Medicine, University of Cambridge, Cambridge CB3 0ES, UK
b St John's College, Cambridge CB3 0ES, UK
* Department of Veterinary Medicine, University of Cambridge, St John's College, Cambridge CB3 0ES, UK.
E-mail address: doctordlwilliams@aol.com

Vet Clin Exot Anim 12 (2009) 1–9
doi:10.1016/j.cvex.2008.11.001
1094-9194/08/$ – see front matter © 2009 Published by Elsevier Inc.

vetexotic.theclinics.com

to move hemolymph around the body cavity; while the cephalopods have complex arterial and venous systems, with a systemic heart consisting of a ventricle enclosed within the walls on the renal sacs without a true pericardial cavity, together with two branchial hearts supplying circulation to the gills.

It is not unusual for invertebrates to have more than one pumping system. Indeed, while hemolymph movement is primarily caused by contractions of the dorsal heart tube in primitive arthropods, this may be supplemented by the action of one of a large number of accessory hearts. Note, for instance, the pumping systems in the legs of insects, such as the cricket and locust, where the pretarsus flexor has been recruited as a contractile element to move hemolymph,[1] providing the oxygen for rapid muscle contraction. Mention should also be made of the wing-heart pumping system in Lepidoptera and Colleoptera where a diaphragm pumping system, derived not from the myocardium but from segmental muscle, allows generation of high pressures of hemolymph to keep the wing membrane erect. Another structure needing to be kept erect is the long ovipositor of the cricket, where the ovipositor muscles pump countercurrent flows of hemolymph into sinuses to keep this long narrow tube turgid. In each of these cases, specific hemodynamic requirements are fulfilled by these accessory pulsatile organs where systemic circulation would undoubtedly fail.

The systemic circulation has a different function; it moves the hemolymph through the body. This can involve arteries and veins in more advanced species with closed circulatory systems but, in contradistinction, often entails movement of fluid through the coelom in invertebrates with an open circulatory system. In the open systems, the ostia of the heart gather hemolymph from the coelom and the heart tube pumps the fluid forward. In closed systems, the circulation runs through arteries and veins from the heart to the tissues and back to it. We said that the heart pumps the fluid forward, yet in many cases changes in direction have a physiologic importance. Periodic heartbeat reversal is important in many arthropods not because of circulatory requirements but because of tracheal ventilation. Moving hemolymph between the anterior and posterior body compartments allows alternating tracheal ventilation. Anatomic and physiologic adaptations range from novel anterior and caudal valved openings in the heart tube, to differential pulse rates for anteriograde and retrograde flows linking with varying diastolic filling in different species with diverse circulatory anatomies. Hemolymph flow may not necessarily involve a single dorsal heart tube. The leech heart, a well-studied system, involves not one dorsal vessel but two lateral ones, generated from segmental modules.[2] Why two hearts beating in synchrony? One produces peristaltic waves with pressures of 50 mm Hg, while the other beats at a much lower pressure of around 20 mm Hg, probably providing segmental circulation, while the high-pressure heart pumps blood forward for locomotor activity. Each heart can pump at either pressure and the switching between the two activities is precipitous and controlled by the nervous system; which is the subject of considerable experimental work.

The heart may also be differentiated with regard to its source of electrical rhythmicity. Some invertebrate species have myogenic hearts, in which electrical activity originates in the heart muscle itself, as in invertebrates as diverse as the primitive crustacean *Triops,* in which the heart is merely a longitudinal tube,[3] and the more advanced snails, such as *Aplysia,* with hearts differentiated into an auricle and ventricle.[4] Others, such as the lobster, have neurogenic hearts, in which the rhythmic discharge of motor neurons, from the cardiac ganglion on the inner dorsal surface of the heart, produce the heartbeat. For myogenic initiation of the heartbeat, two essential physiologic factors are central: a pacemaker must be present either as a specific center, a part of the muscle itself or an inherent function of the muscle as a whole.

Electrocardiograms of insect hearts generally show smooth waveforms typical of myogenically stimulated hearts. Isolated myocardial fibers have classical pacemaker characteristics associated with Ca^{2+} influx through L-type calcium channels and a decrease in K^+ conductance–Na^+ and Cl^- channels appear not to be of any importance. Myogenically initiated cardiac activity depends on electrical coupling of all cardiac cells to one another. Gap junctions are a relatively recent evolutionary advance; most invertebrates have what is known as low-ohm junctions, which have similar properties.[5]

INVERTEBRATE MODELS OF ABNORMAL CARDIAC ORGANOGENESIS

Two invertebrates used as models of cardiac organogenesis are the fruit fly, *Drosophila melanogaster,* and the ascidian sea squirt, *Ciona intestinalis. Ciona* is a member of the tunicates, a group of sessile marine invertebrates. While they appear exceptionally primitive (**Fig. 1**), these animals are chordates, and thus very close cousins of the vertebrates.[6] Three important chordate characteristics are seen in *Ciona* tadpole larva: a dorsal hollow nerve cord, the notochord, and a postanal tail. Once the organism has attached to its substrate, the tail and other chordate structures are resorbed while rudiments in the tadpole head differentiate into adult organs, including the heart. The simplicity of the organism makes it ideal as a model system. Gastrulation is initiated when the organism is only at a 110 cell stage and the fully formed tadpole larva contains less than 3000 cells. In even the simplest vertebrate embryo, gastrulation occurs in the context of tens to hundreds of thousands of cells and the earliest fetal stage is made up of millions of cells. The genetic basis of these tunicates is similarly much less complex than vertebrates, but even so, the genetic pathways of *Ciona* development are remarkably well conserved between these protochordates and higher vertebrates.

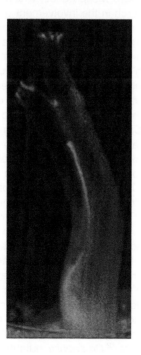

Fig. 1. Ciona the sea squirt.

The tunicate heart is a simple, single-compartment organ located ventrally just posterior to the pharynx and anterior to the stomach. It is a valveless myocardial tube encased in a pericardial coelom. This tube is V-shaped and fits into a triangular pericardial sac. The myocardial cells are epithelial with striated myofilaments luminally and nuclei are situated near the pericardium. Excitation–contraction coupling occurs through junctions similar to the intercalated discs of the vertebrate myocardium.[7] The *Ciona* heart lacks a defined endocardium but has a luminal lining consisting of the basal lamina of the myoepithelial cells. The junction of these myocardial and pericardial cells comprises a dense extracellular matrix, known as the raphe, and at either end of the heart tube is a ring of small cells and an area known as the growth zone. The *Ciona* heart grows throughout life is this area. Large vessels at either end of the heart branch out to form a plexus of smaller vessels throughout the body. The heart drives blood through these vessels by peristalsis. The striated myofibrils form a tight spiral around the heart tube, so that the pumping action is rather a wringing of blood through the tube. A similar anatomy and physiologic organization of pumping is seen in the embryo zebrafish heart.[8]

The key question in using the *Ciona* heart as a model for vertebrate cardiac development and physiology is whether there is indeed a link between this single-chambered heart tube and the multi-chambered mammalian heart. The amniote heart of the mammal, reptile, and bird, is constructed from at least two so-called heart fields. The left ventricle and atrial chambers arise from one primary field, while the right ventricle, its outflow tract and atrial chamber, derive from a secondary heart field which comes from the pharyngeal mesoderm. The chordate heart is equivalent to the first of these two embryonic heart fields. Heart development in *Ciona* involves a set of transcription factors also seen in the organogenesis of the vertebrate heart. Mesp is a basic-helix-loop-helix transcription factor, which is central in early cardiac development. Mammals have two Mesp genes; which is a typical gene duplication that somewhat confuses research in the involvement of these genes. More primitive organisms, such as *Ciona*, demonstrate genetic forms prior to such gene duplication. There is one Mesp gene in this species called Ci-Mesp, and it is expressed specifically in precardiac lineage cells; while Mesp1 and Mesp2, in the mouse, have many effects in determining Notch signaling in the paraxial mesoderm. Mesp knockout mice do not proceed to gastrulation, making analysis of Mesp involvement in cardiac development impossible. Ci-Mesp knockout *Ciona* have specifically disrupted heart development (**Fig. 2**).[9] Use of the Mesp enhancer gene to promote cardiac development resulted in an ectopic heart in treated *Ciona* by directly activating a second transcription factor Ets1/2 which makes precardiac lineage cells responsive to fibroblast growth factor, thus giving a markedly expanded group of precursor cardiac cells.

Mesp is also a key inducer of cardiac development in vertebrates through changes in *Dkk-1* and Wnt signaling.[10] This may prove very important in the cardiac differentiation of human stem cells for cardiac myocyte regeneration; using biomarkers to select suitable cells may allow selection of cardiogenic cells from within a pluripotent stem cell pool.[11]

A second key gene in cardiac development is tinman (tin), which is seen as a number of homologues in vertebrates but one single gene in *Ciona* and *Drosophila*. Tin was the first homeodomain transcriptional factor demonstrated in any organism, making mesodermal cells respond to signals inducing cardiac development. It encourages potential cardioblasts to develop into myoblasts with contractile fibrils by upregulating several other genes and thus acting as a lynch pin in the genetic control of cardiac development. The vertebrate homologue of tinman is *Nkx2-5,* a key homeobox gene in mammalian cardiac development.[12] *Drosophila* mutants lacking tinman fail to develop

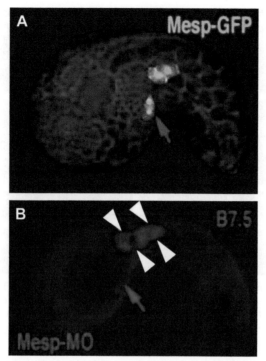

Fig. 2. Mesp expression in wild-type Ciona (A) and lack of expression and subsequent cardiac development in Mesp knock-out Ciona (B). (*From* Davidson B. Ciona intestinalis as a model for cardiac development. Semin Cell Dev Biol 2007;18:16–26; with permission.)

their dorsal cardiac myotube while mice homozygous for a mutant of *Nkx2-5* are characterized by small deformed hearts. Heterozygous mutations in the gene have been linked to atrial and ventricular septal defects, tetralogy of Fallot and Ebstein's tricuspid valve anomaly.[13] Ectopic expression of tinman, on the other hand, increases numbers of cardioblasts in *Drosophila* embryos (**Fig. 3**).[14] Whether they are involved in cardiac abnormalities in any species of veterinary relevance has yet to be determined, while the *Nkx2-5* has been isolated and characterized in the dog.[15]

Third, the Hox genes, long known to be master controllers of segment identity in organisms such as the fruit fly *Drosophila,* and in organogenesis, in more advanced organisms, such as mammals, have a pivotal role in cardiac development. The *Drosophila* myotube is known to consist of 52 pairs of myoendothelial cells forming the heart and aorta. As might be expected from their role in segmental organization, the Hox genes are vital in the axial patterning of the *Drosophial* heart tube. The four homeotic genes Antennapaedia (*Antp*), Ultrabithorax (*Ubx*), abdominal-A (*abd-A*), and abdominal-B (*abd-B*) are sequentially expressed in a nonoverlapping form in the cardiac myotube. Hox-dependent myodiversification is important in defining the morphogenesis of the *Drosophila* heart, a feature also seen in more advanced cardiac organogenesis.

Homozygous Hox-A1 mutations disrupt, not only cardiac development in mammals, but also brainstem and inner ear development.[16] Bosley-Saluh-Alorainy syndrome and Athabascan brainstem dysgenesis often involves congenital cardiac disease, specifically with abnormalities of the left ventricular outflow tract as well as these other

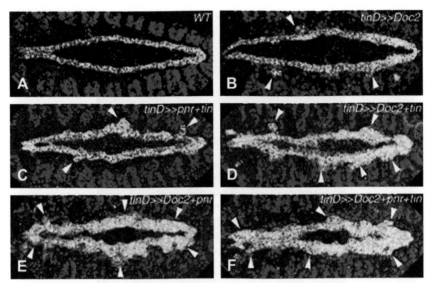

Fig. 3. Increasing tinman expression from images (*A*), wild-type, to (*F*) yields additional cardioblasts (*arrows*). (*From* Zafran S, Reim I, Qian L, et al. Cardioblast-intrinsic tinman activity controls proper diversification and differentiation of myocardial cells in Drosophila. Development 2006;133:4073–83; and *Courtesy of* M. Frasch, PhD, New York, NY; with permission.)

non-cardiac anomalies.[17] This illustrates the wide fields of influence of these primitive organizational genes.

INVERTEBRATE MODELS OF GENETIC FACTORS IN CARDIAC AGEING

Having examined the opportunities the invertebrate heart can give for study of normal and abnormal cardiac development, we turn to the other end of life, that of cardiac ageing. Here the simplicity of these invertebrate genomes again allows dissection of the roles played by various genes in cardiac ageing. Ion channels such as those encoded by the genes *KCNQ* and *HERG* are vital in normal heart function in animals from fruit flies to humans and mutations herein can lead to arrythmia and cardiomyopathies in just such diverse species.[18] *KCNQ* encodes a key potassium channel responsible for repolarization of the cardiac action potential, and thus, mutations in *Drosophila* lead to perturbation of the normal heart function (**Fig. 4**) as in mammals from mice to man.[19] These changes mimic the alterations in cardiac function seen in aging. Survival of these fruit flies is not tightly linked to their cardiac function, so they can be used as a model for gradually decreasing cardiac health.

A key feature of the aging heart in any organism is the maximum heart rate achievable under stress, this being seen both in the fruit fly and in man. The *Drosophila* SUR gene (*dSUR*), encoding a subunit of the ATP-sensitive potassium channel, dramatically decreases in expression in the aging fruit fly heart, while *d*SUR knockout in young fruit fly hearts yields responses to external pacing-induced stress indistinguishable from older hearts.[20]

It is not just cardiac-specific genes that are important in heart aging however. Insulin-like growth factor (*IGF*) signaling, a well-known pathway regulating longevity, protects *Drosophila* hearts from decreases in resting heart rate and increases in heart failure through pacing-induced stress, two well-recognized effects of cardiac aging.[21]

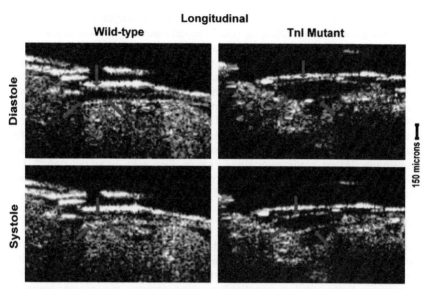

Fig. 4. Cardiac dimensions as measured by optical coherence tomography in wild-type and troponin-mutant Drosophila. (*From* Wolf MJ, Amrein H, Izatt JA, et al. Drosophila as a model for the identification of genes causing adult human heart disease. Proc Natl Acad Sci USA 2006;103:1394–9; with permission. Copyright © 2006, National Academy of Sciences, USA.)

Changes in *IGF* signaling may be related to changes in oxidative stress, given the upregulation in *dFOXO* in such animals. Nevertheless, *Chico,* mutants with extended lifespan associated with *IGF* alterations, do not have increased resistance to oxidative stress and, as in many of these situations, numerous pathways to reduced senescence may be at work.

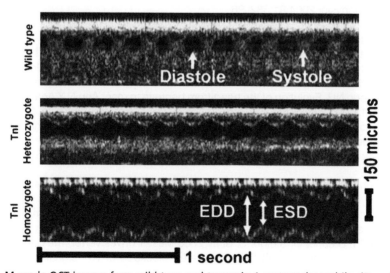

Fig. 5. M-mode OCT images from wild-type and troponin 1 mutant drosophila. (*From* Wolf MJ, Amrein H, Izatt JA, et al. Drosophila as a model for the identification of genes causing adult human heart disease. Proc Natl Acad Sci USA 2006;103:1394–9; with permission. Copyright © 2006, National Academy of Sciences, USA.)

Two other key genes in cardiac biology are troponin and dystrophin. Recent work using optical coherence tomography (OCT), which measures backscattered light as a function of depth and thus provides subsurface imaging with spatial resolution in the region of 10 μm, has allowed detailed evaluation of heart structure and function in troponin 1 mutants with cardiomyopathy.[22] Flies with mutations in sarcomeric contractile proteins such as hdpl2 were generated from mutagenesis experiments which yielded flies with abnormal flight. These homozygous *Tn1* mutants had enlarged heart chambers on diastole (**Figs. 4** and **5**) and markedly impaired systolic function. The heterozygote genotype yielded a partially dominant effect with impaired systolic function but normal diastolic dimensions. *Drosophila,* with a mutation in tropomyosin 2, similarly have dilated cardiomyopathy,[23] as do flies with δ-sarcoglycan.[24] These mutants go to show how valuable studies on the invertebrate heart can be, allowing evaluation at a most basic level, to cardiac biology and disease.

SUMMARY

The content of this article may not be what many readers were expecting when confronted by the title "Cardiac biology and disease in invertebrates," but the author hopes that this discussion of the genetic dissection of cardiac development, disease, and aging, when using these primitive, genetically simple organisms, may provide some interesting avenues for further consideration and research among veterinarians who might not have previously considered that such simple organisms, as sea squirts or fruit flies, could provide any interest with regard to their cardiac biology.

REFERENCES

1. Hantschk A. Functional morphology of accessory circulatory organs in the legs of Hemiptera. Int J Insect Morphol Embryol 1991;20:259–73.
2. Wenning A, Cymbalyuk GS, Calabreses RL. Heartbeat control in leeches. 1 constriction pattern and neural modulation of blood pressure in intact animals. J Neurophysiol 2004;91:382–96.
3. Yamagishi H, Ando H, Makioka T. Myogenic heartbeat in the primitive crustacean triops longicaudatus. Biol Bull 1997;193:350–8.
4. Buckett KJ, Peters M, Benjamin PR. Excitation and inhibition of the heart of the snail, lymnaea, by non-FMRFamidergic motoneurons. J Neurophysiol 1990;63: 1436–47.
5. Bishopric NH. Evolution of the heart from bacteria to man. Ann N Y Acad Sci 2005; 1047:13–29.
6. Delsuc F, Brinkman H, Phillippe H. 2006 Phylogenomics and the reconstruction of the tree of life. Nat Rev Genet 2005;6(5):361–75.
7. Lorber V, Rayns DG. Cellular junctions in the tunicate heart. J Cell Sci 1972;10: 211–27.
8. Forouhar AS, Leibling M, Hickerson A, et al. The embryonic vertebrate heart tube is a dynamic suction pump. Science 2006;312:751–3.
9. Davidson B. 2007 Ciona intestinalis as a model for cardiac development. Semin Cell Dev Biol 2007;18:16–26.
10. David R, Brenner C, Steiber S, et al. 2008 MesP1 drives vertebrate cardiovascular differentiation through Dkk-1-mediated blockade of Wnt-signalling. Nat Cell Biol 2008;10(3):338–45.
11. Nelson TG, Faustino RS, Chiriac A, et al. 2008 CXCR4+/FLK-1+ biomarkers select a cardiopoietic lineage from embryonic stem cells. Stem Cells 2008; 26(6):1464–73.

12. Xavier-Neto J, Castro RA, Sampaio AC, et al. Simões-Costa MS parallel avenues in the evolution of hearts and pumping organs. Cell Mol Life Sci 2007;64:719–34.
13. Benson DW, Silberbach GM, Kavanaugh-McHugh A, et al. Mutations in the cardiac transcription factor NKX2.5 affect diverse cardiac developmental pathways. J Clin Invest 1999;104:1567–73.
14. Zaffran S, Reim I, Qian L, et al. Cardioblast-intrinsic tinman activity controls proper diversification and differentiation of myocardial cells in Drosophila. Development 2006;133:4073–83.
15. Hyun C, Lavulo L, O'Leary C. Isolation and characterization of the canine NKX2-5 gene. J Anim Breed Genet 2006;123:213–6.
16. Tischfield MA, Bosley TM, Salih MA, et al. Homozygous HOXA1 mutations disrupt human brainstem, inner ear, cardiovascular and cognitive development. Nat Genet 2005;37:1035–7.
17. Bosley TM, Alorainy IA, Salih MA, et al. The clinical spectrum of homozygous HOXA1 mutations. Am J Med Genet A 2008;146A:1235–40.
18. Ocorr K, Perrin L, Lim HY, et al. Genetic control of heart function and aging in Drosophila. Trends Cardiovasc Med 2007;17(5):177–82.
19. Ocorr K, Reeves NL, Wessells RJ, et al. KCNQ potassium channel mutations cause cardiac arrhythmias in Drosophila that mimic the effects of aging. Proc Natl Acad Sci U S A 2007;104:3943–8.
20. Akasaka T, Klinedinst S, Ocorr K, et al. The ATP-sensitive potassium (KATP) channel-encoded dSUR gene is required for Drosophila heart function and is regulated by tinman. Proc Natl Acad Sci U S A 2006;103:11999–2004.
21. Wessells RJ, Fitzgerald E, Cypser JR, et al. Insulin regulation of heart function in aging fruit flies. Nat Genet 2004;36(12):1275–81.
22. Wolf MJ, Amrein H, Izatt JA, et al. Drosophila as a model for the identification of genes causing adult human heart disease. Proc Natl Acad Sci U S A 2006;103(5):1394–9.
23. Taghli-Lamallem O, Akasaka T, Hogg G, et al. Dystrophin deficiency in Drosophila reduces lifespan and causes a dilated cardiomyopathy phenotype. Aging Cell 2008;7(2):237–49, Epub 2008 Jan 23.
24. Allikian MJ, Bhabha G, Dospoy P, et al. Reduced life span with heart and muscle dysfunction in Drosophila sarcoglycan mutants. Hum Mol Genet 2007;16(23):2933–43.

Fish Cardiovascular Physiology and Disease

Johanna Sherrill, DVM, MS[a], E. Scott Weber III, VMD, MSc[b],*,
Gary D. Marty, DVM, PhD[c,d],
Stephen Hernandez-Divers, BVetMed, DZooMed, MRCVS[e]

KEYWORDS

- Fish • Cardiac • Cardiovascular
- Fish cardiovascular physiology • Fish heart
- Fish heart disease • Fish cardiac pathologic conditions

The cardiovascular system of a fish is uniquely suited to aquatic vertebrate life. Adaptation strategies for the lifestyle and environment of fish can result in distinctive interspecific variations of cardiovascular physiology. For example, highly migratory and pelagic bluefin tuna (*Thunnus thynnus*) have an unusual adaptation in which blood temperature in the heart can be several degrees cooler than in other parts of the body, such as skeletal muscle.[1] The warmer muscles have higher contraction rates and increased activity[1] to support greater swimming speeds and power. The bluefin tuna can also maintain a more stable core body temperature, in contrast to true poikilothermic fish (body temperature equal to that of ambient water), which may allow for range expansion of these tuna into temperate environs.[1]

Fish patients with cardiovascular disorders present a challenge in terms of diagnostic evaluation and therapeutic options; however, the clinician can approach these cases in fish using similar methods to those employed for other companion animals. Pharmacokinetic and treatment data in fish are limited, especially with regard to specific clinical syndromes, such as cardiovascular disease. As a result, drug types and dosages used in fish are largely empiric.[2] Clinicians who evaluate and treat fish in private, aquarium, zoologic, or aquaculture settings need to rely on sound clinical judgment after thorough historical and physical evaluation.

[a] PO Box 157, Pacific Grove, CA 93950, USA
[b] Companion Avian and Exotic Animal Service, Department of Aquatic Animal Health, University of California, Medicine and Epidemiology, 2108 Tupper Hall, Davis, CA 95616–8747, USA
[c] Department of Anatomy, Physiology, and Cell Biology, University of California, School of Veterinary Medicine, Davis, CA 95616, USA
[d] Ministry of Agriculture and Lands, Animal Health Centre, 1767 Angus Campbell Road, Abbotsford, British Columbia V3G 2M3, Canada
[e] Zoological Medicine, Department of Small Animal Medicine and Surgery, College of Veterinary Medicine, University of Georgia, Athens, GA 30602, USA
* Corresponding author.
E-mail address: epweber@ucdavis.edu (E.S. Weber).

Vet Clin Exot Anim 12 (2009) 11–38
doi:10.1016/j.cvex.2008.08.002
1094-9194/08/$ – see front matter © 2009 Elsevier Inc. All rights reserved.

Fish cardiovascular anatomy, physiology, diagnostic evaluation, monitoring, common diseases, cardiac pathologic conditions, and formulary options are presented with the goal of providing veterinarians involved in fish medicine with clinically relevant tools. The references collected for this issue are of particular utility for more advanced applications.

TELEOST CARDIOVASCULAR ANATOMY

Although more than 53,000 species and subspecies of fishes are documented, this issue describes the general teleost or bony fish cardiovascular system, because this is the largest and most common class of fish encountered by veterinarians. Although many variations and alterations of the general teleost scheme can occur, in most fish, the heart is surrounded by the pharynx (dorsally), pectoral girdle (ventrally and laterally), and liver (caudally) (**Fig. 1**). Heart chambers and blood flow are histologically illustrated in **Fig. 2**.

Components

Fish cardiovascular system components operate together to support these poikilothermic vertebrates adapted to an aquatic environment. The fish cardiovascular system consists of a four-chambered heart arranged in series (see **Fig. 2**); arteries, veins, arterioles, and capillaries; nucleated erythrocytes, thrombocytes (no platelets), and leukocytes; lymphatics and reticuloendothelial tissue; and neural, endocrine, and paracrine tissues or receptors. The cardiovascular system in fish functions primarily to facilitate distribution of blood throughout the body for cellular exchange of gases, electrolytes, inorganic ions, organic products, and nutrients; to augment the removal of waste materials from cells; and to play active and passive roles in fish immunology.

In general, the heart of a fish is composed of elastic tissue and cardiac muscle, similar to a mammal. In most species, the four-chambered heart receives deoxygenated blood from the hepatic and paired common cardinal veins (ducts of Cuvier) into the first cardiac chamber, the sinus venosus. The sinus venosus is a thin-muscled contractile compartment that is ill defined, except by its separation from the next compartment, the atrium, by a sinoatrial valve at the sinoatrial junction. The next compartment is the atrium, which is thin walled, muscular, reticular, and contractile. Blood passes through the atrium into the heavily muscled ventricle through the atrioventricular (AV) junction, achieving unidirectional blood flow as a result of paired AV valves. The ventricle in fish is single chambered and composed of an inner layer called the

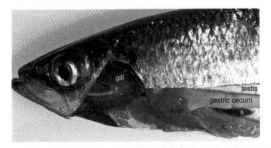

Fig.1. The heart (*arrows*) in this Pacific herring (*Clupea pallasii*) is surrounded by the gill, pectoral girdle (pg, cut away), and lobes of the liver (L). Other visceral structures include the testis, gastric cecum, spleen (s), intestine (i), and intestinal ceca (ic). Anisakid nematode parasites are coiled on the surface of the liver and intestinal ceca.

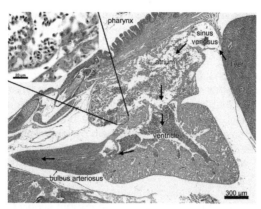

Fig. 2. Normal heart of a juvenile sablefish (*Anoploma fimbria*). Unoxygenated blood flows through the sinus venosus, atrium, ventricle, and bulbus arteriosus on its way to the gills for oxygenation. The green box outlines the area shown in detail in inset (*upper left*). Hematoxylin and eosin stain.

spongiosa and an outer layer called the compacta. The ratio of spongiosa to compacta varies based on the species. Most bony fish have little if any compacta layer unless they are strongly pelagic, whereas many shark species (elasmobranchs or cartilaginous fish) have a thick compacta that may comprise up to 40% of ventricular mass.[3] Blood is then pumped by way of the ventricle through another pair of valves at the ventricular-bulbar junction into the bulbus arteriosus. In teleosts, the bulbus arteriosus is composed of noncontractile elastic tissue. In sharks, this compartment is called the conus arteriosus and has a thin wall of contractile cardiac muscle marked by several transverse rows of valves.[4] The deoxygenated blood then flows from the bulbus arteriosus into the ventral aorta.

Blood

The blood cells in fish are similar to those of other vertebrates and consist of erythrocytes, thrombocytes, and leukocytes. The erythrocytes are nucleated, oval, and range in size from 9 μm in diameter for hagfish (class Myxina) to 36 μm long in lungfish (subclass Dipnoi).[5] Fish leukocytes consist of lymphocytes, granulocytes, and monocytes (macrophages). Most macrophages stay fixed in the tissues and rarely circulate in the blood. The reticuloendothelial system of the atrium is a major site for pathogen recognition and destruction by antigen-presenting cells and fixed macrophages. In some species of fish, phagocytic cells on the heart endothelial cells function in cardiac-based host defense.[6] Unlike in mammals, no hematopoiesis occurs in the bone marrow. In fish, hematopoiesis occurs in a variety of organs, including the anterior kidney, spleen, liver, thymus, and gut mesodermal tissue. In sturgeon, pericardial and meningeal foci of hematopoiesis are normal and should not be confused with epicarditis or meningitis.

The circulating blood volume of fish varies from 3% to 6.6% of the body weight, depending on the species.[7] Although hematocrits can vary greatly, most teleosts have hematocrits ranging from 20% to 30%.[8]

Different hemoglobin compositions exist in fish to facilitate environmental adaptation.[5] Notothenioids (Antarctic icefishes) are adapted to live in extremely cold waters through the use of antifreeze blood proteins and a highly sedentary lifestyle.[9] Because frigid water is oxygen rich, some less active icefishes lack hemoglobin in their blood and can supply the body with oxygen using only blood plasma.[9]

Blood Vessels and General Circulation in Fish

Apart from a few distinctions, the vessels containing and transporting blood in fish are analogous to vessels in other vertebrates. Fish have two main types of arteries: thick-walled afferent vessels that lead away from the heart to the gills and thinner-walled efferent vessels that lead away from the gills to the body. In some species of fish, the dorsal aorta may have primitive pumps to help peripheral circulation. As in other vertebrates, veins return blood to the heart and the heart itself is fed by coronary arteries. Compared with mammals, capillaries in fish are more permeable and do not have an osmotic gradient.

The circulatory pattern in most teleosts is quite basic. After leaving the gills, the dorsal aorta anteriorly divides into paired carotid arteries that supply the head and brain. Posteriorly, the dorsal aorta remains a single vessel and becomes the caudal artery that courses through the ventral hemal arches of the vertebrae. Arteries, which include the branchial, celiac, mesenteric, ovarian, spermatic, renal, gastric, parietal, renal, and iliac arteries, branch off of the dorsal aorta and caudal artery to provide oxygenated blood to the gills and coelomic organs. Segmental arteries supply blood to the fins and the musculature.

Venous return largely depends on the caudal vein, which lies just ventral to the caudal artery, protected by the hemal arches. This is the main vessel used for phlebotomy in most species of fish. In many species of cartilaginous and bony fish, return circulation requires caudal pumps or hearts with valves, which are augmented by swimming activity and lateral movement of the caudal peduncle.[8] Blood returns by way of segmental, caudal, renal, hepatic, common cardinal, subintestinal, abdominal, anterior cardinal, and branchial veins.

Several anatomic patterns of venous return in various fish species have been documented.[10] Although the physiologic significance and importance of these anatomic variations is unknown in teleosts, many species of fish, such as koi (*Cyprinus carpio*), have venous return from segmental veins through a renal or hepatic portal system, which may have profound pharmacokinetic effects on therapeutics administered at caudal intramuscular sites.[10] Theoretically, if pharmacologic agents are administered in areas that the segmental veins are draining directly through the renal portal or hepatic portal systems, these agents may be processed by the kidney or liver, respectively, before being systemically circulated, resulting in a loss of active drug or possible toxic effects on the kidney or liver.

Fish also have a secondary circulation in parallel to the primary circulatory system consisting of small arteriole-like vessels.[11] Although the use and function of this secondary circulation are still not fully understood, many hypothesize that these vessels may be part of the lymphatics.[12] The concept of a fish lymphatic system was first introduced in 1769.[13] Later, researchers identified a network of lymphatics associated with gastrointestinal tissues and the dermis.[14] Recent research in zebrafish identified vessels in fish similar to lymphatic vessels in mammals, distinct from arterioles and the venous circulation.[15]

Cardiac Physiology and Mechanics

In the aquatic environment, several challenges must be overcome to maximize cardiovascular efficiency. The function of the fish cardiovascular system is influenced by the following factors: fish have hydrodynamic rather than gravitational pressures exerted on them while in water; fish are ectotherms (absorbing heat from their environs to maintain body temperature) and poikilotherms, whose physiologic functions are influenced by environmental temperature; and finally, aquatic environments are relatively oxygen poor compared with terrestrial environments and are subject to Raoult's law (the vapor pressure of a solution is proportional to the number of molecules per unit volume in the solution).

Notably, the heart of a fish does not pump oxygenated blood like the heart of a mammal. Instead, the fish heart pumps only deoxygenated blood to the gills for respiration. Blood enters the ventral aorta, travels through afferent branchial arteries to the gill arches, achieves gas exchange when passing through capillary beds, and then returns as oxygenated blood by way of efferent branchial arteries into the dorsal aorta.

Blood Pressure

Blood pressure measurement is not practical for routine determination in clinical fish patients. In the research setting, however, dorsal and ventral aortic pressures are studied in detail by fish physiologists using direct methods.[12] For example, in resting rainbow trout maintained at 11°C, researchers recorded ventral and dorsal aortic pressures of 39 mm Hg and 31 mm Hg, respectively.[12]

Cardiac Morphology and Output

Fish cardiac morphology and cardiac innervation have been reviewed.[16] The gross shape of the heart ventricle in selected fish species can vary from tubular to saccular to pyramidal, with the latter being the more structurally efficient shape for pumping **(Fig. 3)**.[17,18] Ultrastructural morphology of the fish heart, including the AV valve, endocardium, and myocardium, can be quite different among species.[17,19]

Cardiac output is governed by heart rate and stroke volume. Mechanisms for increasing cardiac output differ between fish and most vertebrates.[20] Mammals, birds, and reptiles increase their cardiac output through large increases in heart rate paired with smaller increases in stroke volume, whereas fish use marked increases in stroke volume and only modest changes in heart rate.[21]

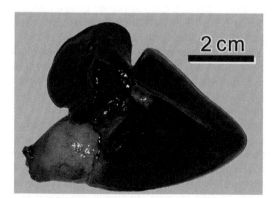

Fig. 3. View of the heart of an adult bluefin tuna (*Thunnus thynnus*) shows a pyramidal shape of the ventricle. The atrium is above on the left, and the distinct white fibrous bulbous arteriosus is located next to the ventricle on the left. The bulbus arteriosus is analogous to the aorta in mammals and is composed of abundant elastic connective tissue. (*Adapted from* Tuna Research and Conservation Center, Stanford University archives, Stanford University, CA; with permission.)

Innervation and Pacemaker Activity

Cranial nerve X innervates the heart in most groups of fish, and parasympathetic fibers are largely inhibitory, slowing heart rate and activity when activated.[21] The site and size of the pacemaker region in different species of fish are variable, but for most species, the heart beat is initiated at the sinoatrial node.[22] For example, sinoatrial pacemaker tissue is located at the sinoatrial valve base in the rainbow trout (*Oncorhyncus mykiss*) heart.[23] In one study, the intrinsic rate of the sinoatrial pacemaker studied in vitro was higher in rainbow trout hearts acclimated to colder temperatures versus those kept at warmer water temperatures.[23]

Environmental Influences on Fish Cardiovascular Physiology

Fish heart rates can vary with temperature as a compensatory mechanism. In general, coldwater fish in water temperatures of 5°C to 11°C have a heart rate of 15 to 30 beats per minute, whereas warm-water fish (19°C–24°C) can have a heart rate of 30 to 50 beats per minute.[12] Some species, such as the yellowfin tuna, *Thunnus albacares*, have heart rates as high as 96 beats per minute (at 26°C).[12]

Cardiac contractility must be maintained despite exposure to changing water temperature and acidity level. Intensive rearing methods in aquaculture can alter oxygen content, temperature, pH, and other factors that lead to stress on the cardiac function of resident fish.[24] Different fish species can tolerate a wide range of pH values and temperatures because of myocardial adaptations that preserve contractility.[24]

Insufficient dissolved oxygen levels in the water lead to hypoxia, often reflected by increased gilling rates by resident fish and subsequent respiratory distress.[2] Maintaining 1.5 to 2.0 L/h of air for each liter of aquarium water is recommended at all times.[25] Hypoxia can result in pathologic changes within fish cardiac cells.[26] These effects may be acute, resulting in mortality, or chronic, causing cell damage. Diets rich in polyunsaturated fatty acids of the n-3 type may help fish to resist cardiac tissue damage from chronic hypoxic conditions.[27]

CLINICAL EVALUATION OF CARDIOVASCULAR DISEASE

Evaluating the cardiovascular system of fish in a clinical setting can be challenging for the veterinary practitioner. A primary cardiovascular problem may not be initially suspected when examining a sick fish. Detailed references with suggested diagnostic approaches to fish disease problems are available to veterinarians.[2,10,28–32] As for any exotic animal patient, evaluation of a fish patient might include signalment, history, environmental conditions, clinical signs, visual assessment, physical examination, and necropsy of conspecifics. With few exceptions, suboptimal environmental conditions are a common root cause of lesions in fish. Water quality must be closely monitored and should be the first thing checked when mortalities occur.

A visual examination can be performed with minimal stress and constitutes an important step in evaluating a fish patient.[2,29] Physical examination with diagnostic procedures requires removal of the patient from its aquatic environment, followed by manual or chemical restraint, which is clearly a stressful event for a sick fish. Stress associated with handling of fish patients for diagnostics and sample collection can be minimized with properly applied appropriate anesthesia, however.[2]

History and Clinical Signs

Several investigators have recommended questions for fish veterinarians to consider when taking a history.[10,28,29,32,33] A list of behavioral signs of disease in fish is also available.[28] A thorough historical evaluation might include signalment of affected fish; water quality and tank maintenance record review; animal additions and mortalities; diet and dietary changes; quarantine protocol (or the lack of quarantine); recent or current parasitism or infectious diseases; relevant breeding history; when the onset of symptoms occurred; duration of the problem; appetite, attitude, or activity changes; and any current or recent medications or treatments administered.

Table 1 provides a summary of some potential features of history and clinical signs suggestive or supportive of cardiac disease in a fish patient. Some historical indicators that might signal underlying cardiovascular disease in a fish patient include loss of appetite, decrease in activity level, increased tendency to isolate or hide, change in coloration or loss of vibrancy, irregular swimming patterns, buoyancy problems, lethargy, or sudden death.

Signalment

Signalment generally refers to type or species, age, and gender of the affected fish. The age of the fish patient may increase the potential for cardiac pathologic conditions. In salmonids, sexual maturity has been associated with onset of cardiomyopathy, cartilaginous metaplasia, and coronary vessel disease. Fish gender does not seem to be linked to an increase in the likelihood of cardiac disease.

Environmental Conditions

The ecosystem that wild fish inhabit is delicately balanced. For fish in captivity, optimal conditions are difficult to create and often expensive to maintain. Suboptimal environmental conditions begin a cascade of stress-related untoward events in fish, such as catecholamine and corticosteroid release, immune system compromise, biochemical and hematologic alterations, poor growth, and reduced fecundity.[2,28] Abnormal environmental factors, especially unfavorable water quality parameters, can potentially lead to primary or secondary cardiovascular system disorders. Fish reared under

Table 1	
Historical indicators and clinical signs (by system) consistent with cardiovascular disease in fish	
History	Normal (no signs)
	Abnormal behavior, inactive swimming, lethargy, hiding, anorexia or reduced appetite, slowed weight gain, circulatory disturbance signs, buoyancy problems, piping at the surface (open-mouth breathing), sudden death, group mortalities
System	
Mucous membranes, gills	Pale and blanched (white), hyperemic (red)
Integumentary, scales	Color changes (lighter or darker), elevated scales, ventral skin petechiation, hemorrhagic scales or fins, skin ulcers and erosions
Eyes	Exophthalmia, visual deficits, cloudiness, hyphema
Cardiorespiratory	Changes in heart and respiratory (opercular) rates (increased or decreased), piping
Gastrointestinal (coelom)	Distended coelomic cavity, ascites
Swim bladder	Distention, abnormal buoyancy, loss of equilibrium
Musculoskeletal	Weakness, weight loss, poor body condition, irregular swimming patterns
Neurologic	Depression, obtundation, loss of righting reflex

intensive conditions, including salmonids, may be more prone to cardiovascular disease and cardiac-centered infections.[34,35]

Physical Examination

A visual evaluation initiates the physical examination of a fish.[2] Physical evidence of cardiovascular disease in a fish includes (but is not limited to) pale or hyperemic mucous membranes or gill filaments, hemorrhagic scales or fins, dark coloration or melanocyte changes in the skin, increased or decreased gilling activity (respiratory rate changes), piping at the surface (open-mouth breathing), flared opercula, loss of coordination in swimming or muscle activity, weakness, ascites (**Fig. 4**), elevated or edematous scales, exophthalmia, neurologic changes (eg, impaired righting reflex, erratic behavior), equilibrium imbalances, and intolerance or hypersensitivity to anesthesia.

Diagnostic Tests

Several diagnostic techniques can be used to evaluate the cardiovascular system of a fish patient. Skin scrapings and gill or fin biopsies are easily performed procedures that can augment the diagnosis of many disorders of fish.[2,29,36] Paracentesis, fecal analysis, microbial cultures, and radiology often supplement other diagnostic procedures.[2]

GILL OR FIN CLIP

A fresh preparation of a small piece of gill or fin tissue onto a glass slide with a coverslip over a drop of saline is a simple way to assess certain features related to the cardiovascular system.[33,36] For example, a gill biopsy can reveal gill parasites or other infectious agents, gas emboli from supersaturation of water with gases, epithelial damage from chronic suboptimal water conditions, erythrocyte quality and color, developmental changes, and blood parasites.

IMAGING TECHNIQUES
Radiography

In general, radiography is underused in fish medicine.[28] Taking a radiograph of a fish patient requires removal from its water environment, ideally for about a minute or less in most species. The fish is placed on a radiographic table or cassette, where it must

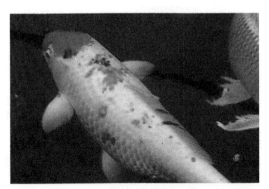

Fig. 4. A koi carp (*Cyprinus carpio*) with coelomic distention attributable to ascites. Differential diagnoses include bacterial sepsis with secondary cardiac disease and failure.

be still enough to allow for proper exposure times to achieve a diagnostic result. This can be done awake in certain amenable species of fish. Anesthesia can be used to decrease unwanted movement and increase yield in diagnostic capability. Mammography cassettes coupled with regular x-ray unit radiation (or refurbished mammography units) can be used to increase the detail and quality of radiographs taken of fish of all sizes. Ascites, swim bladder distention, mass effects, and general organ architecture may be visible on plain films. Unfortunately, specific cardiac detail in a fish is not visualized well using standard or digital radiographic techniques.

Angiography

Angiography, which requires secure and continuous venous access and a fluoroscopy-capable radiology unit, does not seem to be widely used in a clinical veterinary setting for any species, including fish. Angiography would potentially allow detailed visualization of the vasculature and cardiac components of a fish patient.

Ultrasonography (Echocardiography)

Real-time ultrasound of the cardiovascular structures of a fish is potentially a high-yield and low-stress diagnostic modality. The ultrasound probe can be submerged (protected in plastic), and a fish can be scanned while awake and restrained in a small area, holding tank, or even a stretcher.[25,37,38] In the practice setting, ultrasound remains underused, however, perhaps because of the lack of portability of most units and, ultimately, the expense. A portable laptop-type ultrasound unit may be helpful to veterinarians practicing fish medicine. Care must be taken to avoid water damage to the unit or potential dangers arising from mixing electrical power and wet working areas.

Ultrasound can be used to identify and evaluate different heart chambers, real-time blood flow, vascular structures in different locations,[25] and the presence of thrombi in the different chambers or vascular areas of fish, among other conditions. Cardiac myopathy syndrome was diagnosed in vivo in tranquilized submerged Atlantic salmon (*Salmo salar*) using ultrasound.[37] Echocardiograms were performed successfully in multiple shark species as a means of comparing ventricular function.[38] The additional utility of ultrasound in fish includes identification of hepatic parasites, ascites, or coelomic cavity congestion, and different anatomic anomalies.[37]

CT and MRI

The usefulness of CT and MRI in pet or aquarium fish has not been widely explored despite a theoretically excellent yield of information to be gained about cardiovascular anatomy, physiology, pathologic conditions, and function. One disadvantage, apart from access to the unit and associated costs, is that either imaging technique requires inactivity of the fish patient, for at least 5 minutes for an accelerated CT scan and for up to 30 or 40 minutes for an MRI scan, making anesthesia or even euthanasia a requirement. One group used MRI contrast studies to examine environmental adaptational physiology in small teleosts with good results and compared their findings with those of some other studies.[39]

Rigid Endoscopy

Rigid endoscopy provides a minimally invasive technique for the examination of internal structures and can be used to evaluate some important cardiovascular facets of anesthetized fish.[40,41] Although the fish patient must be anesthetized for endoscopy, this diagnostic technique can be performed efficiently and easily in the practice setting. One small incision allows entry of a rigid endoscope into the coelomic cavity and good visualization of many internal structures of the fish patient in addition to collection of body fluids or biopsies using additional endoscopic equipment.

Externally, the endoscope can be positioned under the operculum and into the water streaming over the gills to examine the primary and secondary lamellae. The magnification afforded by the telescope facilitates detailed examination of the secondary lamellae, such that individual erythrocytes can be seen coursing through the capillaries (**Fig. 5**). Coelioscopy permits examination of the internal vasculature associated with various visceral organs. Unfortunately, the heart is typically separated from the coelom by a fibrous membrane, the transverse septum, making direct visualization difficult to impossible. At best, it is possible to perceive diastole and systole through this membrane (**Fig. 6**).

Clinicians with access to a rigid endoscope and appropriate training are encouraged to pursue diagnosis of cardiovascular diseases in fish accordingly. Guides and training courses are readily available for such procedures.[40]

DOPPLER AND PULSE OXIMETRY

A Doppler crystal or probe, such as those used to detect pulses in a small animal, can be placed in several different positions to give an audible and accurate measure of heart rate in an anesthetized fish. Successful areas for Doppler flow probe placement on the fish include the dorsal surface of the tongue, inside the operculum just under the gill arches (gently), or on the ventral surface of the head region over the heart between the pectoral fins (**Fig. 7**).

The use of a pulse oximeter to detect percent oxygen saturation of hemoglobin in the blood is possible in a fish awake or under anesthesia. This method is limited by placement of the sensor clip in a reasonable anatomic location, in which vessels are

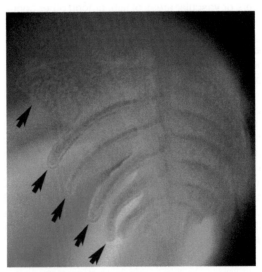

Fig. 5. High magnification (original magnification ×20) view of the tip of a primary gill lamella in a shovelnose sturgeon (*Scaphirhynchus platorynchus*) as seen using a 2.7-mm telescope positioned within the water stream coursing over the gills. Note the numerous secondary lamellae (*arrows*) through which erythrocytes can be seen moving through the capillaries. (*Courtesy of* University of Georgia, College of Veterinary Medicine, Athens, GA; with permission.)

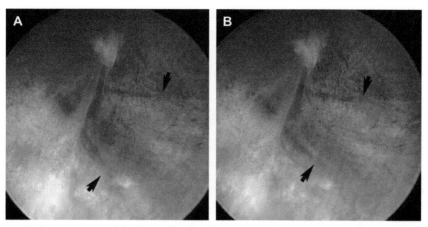

Fig. 6. Endoscopic view of the heart (*outlined by arrows*) of a shovelnose sturgeon (*Scaphirhynchus platorynchus*) as seen from within the cranial coelom using sterile saline insufflation and a 2.7-mm telescope. Note the subtle difference in size and shape between diastole (*A*) and systole (*B*). (*Courtesy of* University of Georgia, College of Veterinary Medicine, Athens, GA; with permission.)

reliably detectable or sufficient to give a reading. The best use of pulse oximetry seems to be for heart beat detection and heart rate monitoring. Placement of an esophageal, rectal, or tongue clip pulse oximeter sensor can result in heart rate measurements that match beats per minute as measured by cardiac ultrasound or Doppler units.

ELECTROCARDIOGRAPHY

Measurement of the electrical activity of the fish heart can be achieved with an electrocardiogram (ECG), commonly used in research experiments.[42,43] Although one cannot use electrical equipment easily in an aquatic environment, attachment of ECG leads to monitor electrical conductivity of the heart of a fish undergoing anesthesia and surgery, such as for celioscopy or celiotomy, is not difficult. Leads are

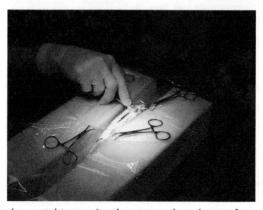

Fig. 7. Use of a Doppler crystal to monitor heart sounds and rate of an anesthetized koi (*Cyprinus carpio*). (*Courtesy of* G. Lewbart, VMD, Raleigh, NC.)

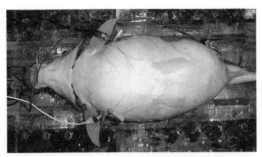

Fig. 8. Placement of ECG leads using the pectoral fins on an anesthetized koi (*Cyprinus carpio*). This method of monitoring cardiac rate and electrical activity is not difficult to perform. Care must be taken when operating electrical equipment in wet environments. (*Courtesy of* A. Klide, VMD, Philadelphia, PA.)

attached using hypodermic needles (usually 25 or 27 gauge) inserted subcutaneously, with one needle placed on each side of the fish between the branchiostegal membrane of the pectoral fins and a third needle placed just caudal to the anus proximal to the caudal peduncle (**Fig. 8**).

Waveforms are analogous to those of other vertebrates, with identifiable P, QRS, and T waves (**Fig. 9**). A P wave occurs after atrial depolarization, followed by a QRS complex signaling ventricular depolarization, and a subsequent T wave marking ventricular repolarization. In the authors' experience, some fish species have produced inconsistent ECG waveforms and an ECG trace that does not reflect expected electroconductivity for a fish. ECGs have been successfully performed in fish and sharks, however, especially in a research setting, often using implanted ECG-recording transmitters.[42–44]

In some species, a "V wave" preceding the P wave occurs and may represent depolarization of the sinus venosus.[12] A "Bd complex" was recorded in a Port

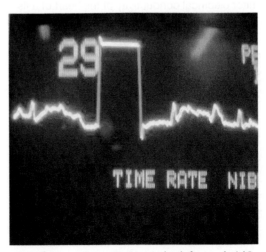

Fig. 9. ECG tracing or waveforms, using a 1-mV standard, from a koi (*Cyprinus carpio*) under anesthesia.

Jackson shark (*Heterodontus portjacksoni*) between the QRS complex and the T wave and was attributed to depolarization of the conus arteriosus.[44] Because the fish heart has intrinsic pacemaker cells that cause the heart to beat long after respiration ceases, ECG waveforms can be detected even after euthanasia using an anesthetic overdose or another physical method listed in the American Veterinary Medical Association (AVMA) guidelines for euthanasia (2007).[45]

CLINICAL PATHOLOGY
Complete Blood Cell Count

Several publications describe methods for bleeding fish of different sizes and handling their blood.[10,29,31,33] Fish blood clots quickly, mandating the collection of blood into preheparinized syringes. Automated complete blood cell count (CBC) machines that are calibrated or developed for mammals cannot be used accurately. Machines that are suitable for the nucleated red blood cells (RBCs) of other animals (eg, birds, reptiles) are useful for fish blood counts. A fresh blood smear onto a glass slide stained with routine trichrome cytology stain is relatively easy to perform, however, and is an accepted means of evaluating fish blood cells and CBCs. Published values of CBCs from certain fish species are available.[10,31,46]

Chemistries

Plasma chemistries in fish are helpful when available, although interpretation is not always clear. This is because of inherent differences among species and a lack of normal data values and ranges for many of the fish species likely to be encountered in a clinical or aquarium setting. Several references list chemistry values to expect in certain fish species.[10,31,46]

NECROPSY EXAMINATION

A thorough postmortem examination is critical to proper assessment of the cardiovascular system of a fish patient. Many excellent fish necropsy guides are available to the veterinary practitioner.[33,36] It may be useful to examine a freshly killed fish or group of fish from an affected tank in addition to any fish found dead to minimize postmortem artifacts, which are especially common in warm-water fish that decompose rapidly after death. Ideally, a complete necropsy is recorded from head to tail, and representative samples are taken from each major organ system, including the heart, bulbus arteriosus, and any large vessels of interest.[33] If any gross lesions, such as defects, cysts, or nodules, are noted on the heart, representative tissue samples should be collected into formalin for histopathologic examination and impression smears should be made for cytologic examination.[28]

CARDIOVASCULAR PATHOLOGIC FINDINGS

Cardiovascular lesions in fish may be primary or secondary to some other cause. A detailed review of all lesions pertaining to the cardiovascular system of fish is beyond the scope of this issue. Descriptive general pathology references are available to fish veterinarians.[47,48] Selected lesions and diseases of the fish heart and vessels that have potential clinical relevance and interest to the veterinary practitioner are summarized in **Table 2**.

Histopathologic examination of the heart, including the bulbus arteriosus, is an important part of any diagnostic necropsy. Because the heart is the only organ that receives blood from the entire body, it often contains microscopic clues, even when

Table 2
Selected causes and lesions associated with or affecting the fish cardiovascular system, including hematopoietic tissues

Cause	Comments	References
Infectious		
Viral		
Alphavirus	Cardiomyopathy syndrome in salmonids; salmon pancreatic disease, heart lesions	34,57
Erythrocytic inclusion body syndrome	Progressive severe anemia in chinook and coho salmon	31
Heart and skeletal muscle inflammation virus	Unknown viral agent; epicarditis, myocarditis, mononuclear cell infiltrates	35,58
Herpesvirus	Channel catfish virus disease, destruction of hematopoietic tissues; exophthalmia, ascites, lethargy, pinpoint hemorrhages at base of fins	31
Iridovirus	Amphophilic inclusion bodies in atrial and ventricular tissues	See Fig. 12
Rhabdovirus	Viral hemorrhagic septicemia virus, endotheliotropic, necrotizing myocarditis; infectious hematopoietic necrosis virus	59
Togavirus	Salmon pancreatic disease; cardiac ventricle compacta tissue necrosis	57
Viral erythrocytic necrosis virus	Unknown viral agent; previously piscine erythrocytic necrosis, intracytoplasmic inclusions in erythrocytes, karyolytic	31
Bacterial	Septicemia can be associated with heart infections, heart failure, thrombus formation in cardiovascular chambers	See Fig. 10
Bacterial kidney disease	*Renibacterium salmoninarum*, salmonids, septic heart failure	60
Furunculosis	*Aeromonas salmonicida*, deep ulcers, many species of fish	31
Mycobacteria	Acid-fast, granulomas in cardiac tissues	61
Nocardia seriolae	Acid-fast bacteria; white nodules in heart of sea bass	62
Streptococcal	*Streptococcus iniae*, gram-positive, inflammation around the heart; erratic swimming, ascites (dropsy), buoyancy disorders	31
Fungal	*Branchiomyces, Exophiala, Ichthyophonus hoferi, Phoma*, or others; opportunistic; tissue invasion; granulomatous inflammation in many marine fish species; hematogenous spread possible	31,63
Saprolegnia or related species	Common in cultured juvenile freshwater fish; invasion from the external surface through the skin	See Fig. 8

Category	Description	Ref
Parasitic	Metazoans (nematodes, trematodes, cestodes), protozoans; cardiac and hematogenous infections	64
Amoebic gill disease	Neoparamoeba spp, gill vascular invasion	31
Contracaecum sp	Atrial tissue nematode larvae invasion; thin-walled atria, damaged muscular trabeculae	64
Henneguya ictaluri	Myxosporidian, within cardiac vessels	65
Myxobolus bulbocordis	Cardiac serosal parasitic cysts	66
Sanguinicola sp	Blood flukes in freshwater fish; eggs virulent to cardiac tissues	
Rickettsial		
Salmon rickettsial disease	Piscirickettsia salmonis, intracellular, gram-negative, common in eastern Pacific cultured salmonids, high mortality rates, decreasing hematocrit, lethargic darkened fish, pale gills	31
Noninfectious		
Congenital/genetic		
Glycogen-storage disease	Distended atria, rounded ventricles	67
Cardiac malformations	Farmed rainbow trout, ventricular hypoplasia in farmed Atlantic salmon	68,69
Degenerative	Sexual maturity in salmonids has been linked to onset of cardiomyopathy, cartilaginous metaplasia, coronary vessel disease	70
	Mineralization of the bulbous arteriosus, adult female rainbow trout	71
Environmental	Suboptimal water quality and environmental conditions can affect cardiovascular health and function	
Increased nitrites	Brown blood disease, methemoglobinemia	31
Water and serum pH levels	Elevation can increase vascular resistance in gill tissues	72
Stress, acute or chronic	Leads to epinephrine release, increased gill permeability, diuresis, coagulopathy, hemoconcentration, decreased growth, compromised immunity, reduced fecundity	2
Idiopathic		
Cardiac lesions	Myocardial and pericardial lesions in farmed halibut; myocardial hypertrophy and karyomegaly in farmed Atlantic salmon	73,74

(continued on next page)

Table 2
(continued)

Cause	Comments	References
Neoplasia	Can occur in cardiovascular structures and tissues; use thorough biopsy and necropsy techniques	33,36
Hemangioendothelial tumors	Bulbous arteriosus, ventricle, gills, vessels; endotheliolomas, hemangiomas, sarcomas; marked epicarditis	75
Mesothelioma	In ventricle, associated with protozoal organisms	76
Nutritional		
Linoleic acid	Atlantic salmon fed high levels (with a low n-3/n-6 ratio) from sunflower oil, thin ventricle walls, myonecrosis	77
Trauma	Superficial lesions can lead to leaky vessels and capillaries, osmotic imbalance, circulatory failure	

a cardiovascular pathologic finding is not the only cause of morbidity. For example, mural thrombi are fairly common in the heart of aquarium fish, with septicemia as the primary differential diagnosis (**Fig. 10**; compare with **Fig. 2**, which demonstrates a normal fish heart).

Rodlet cell endocarditis in the bulbus arteriosus of koi carp is often associated with the intravascular trematode, *Sanguinicola* sp (**Fig. 11**).[49] Koi carp infected with koi herpesvirus, specifically cyprinid herpesvirus-3, sometimes have intranuclear viral inclusions in endothelial cells (see **Fig. 11**). Systemic iridovirus infections have been identified in several fish species (eg, freshwater angelfish [*Pterophyllum scalare*], freshwater discus [*Symphosodon* sp], saltwater Banggai cardinal fish [*Pterapogon kauderni*], saltwater threespine sticklebacks [*Gasterosteus aculeatus*]). Affected fish often have characteristic inclusion bodies in the heart (**Fig. 12**). External fungal infections are common in juvenile freshwater fish; the prognosis is poor when the fungi invade the skin and enter the heart (**Fig. 13**).

ANESTHESIA AND CARDIOVASCULAR MONITORING

Several useful guides for safely and efficiently anesthetizing a fish patient are available to the clinician.[50–52] For example, good results can be achieved in a controlled setting using an easy-to-assemble fish anesthesia machine.[52] Methods for monitoring the cardiovascular system of an anesthetized fish include (but are not limited to) visual observation, ECG (see **Figs. 8** and **9**), Doppler flow crystal (see **Fig. 7**) or probe, ultrasonography, pulse oximetry, and blood gas measurement. Using some of this equipment to monitor sedated or anesthetized fish can prove difficult; as such, ultrasonography is a preferred method for monitoring heart rate and contractility during lengthy diagnostic procedures or surgery.

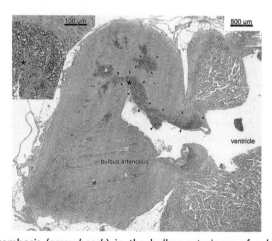

Fig. 10. Mural thrombosis (*arrowheads*) in the bulbus arteriosus of a koi carp (*Cyprinus carpio*) with motile aeromonad septicemia. *Aeromonas veronii* was cultured from the trunk kidney of this fish. The inset demonstrates the details of thrombus (*). Hematoxylin and eosin stain.

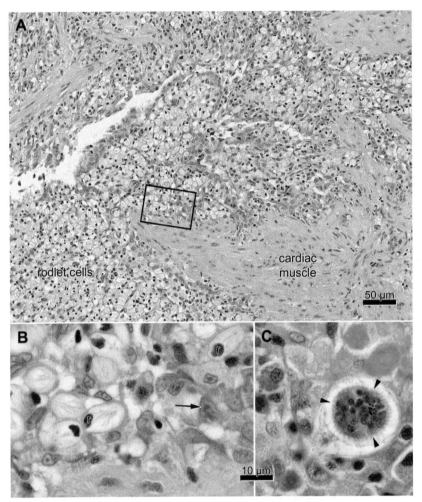

Fig. 11. Tissues from a koi carp (*Cyprinus carpio*) infested with the intravascular trematode *Sanguinicola*; the fish was also positive by polymerase chain reaction for cyprinid herpesvirus-3 (CyHV-3, or koi herpesvirus). (*A*) Bulbus arteriosus with severe rodlet cell endocarditis; black box outlines the area shown in detail in *B*. (*B*) Rodlet cells have an eccentric nucleus (r) and distinctive fibrillar cytoplasm; some endothelial cell nuclei (*arrow*) have amphophilic structures that might be CyHV-3 inclusions. (*C*) Trunk kidney interstitium with a multicellular *Sanguinicola* egg (*arrowheads*), commonly associated with rodlet cell endocarditis. Magnification in *B* and *C* is the same. Hematoxylin and eosin stain.

TREATMENT

Methods to treat fish patients include oral, topical, immersion, and injectable routes of delivery. Immersion methods vary in duration and strength and include dips (less than 15 minutes), baths (more than 15 minutes), flow-through (generally used in aquaculture raceways), and long-term tank treatments (least preferable). Before adding drugs to aquarium water, chemical filtration, such as carbon filters, must be removed, and additional aeration during treatment is advisable.[28]

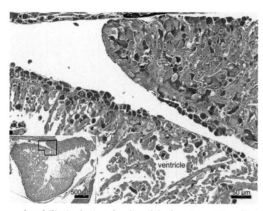

Fig. 12. Abundant amphophilic inclusion bodies (*) characteristic of iridovirus infection in the atrium and ventricle of a threespine stickleback (*Gasterosteus aculeatus*). The black box in the inset outlines the area shown in detail in the rest of the figure. Hematoxylin and eosin stain.

Pharmacokinetic data and established treatment protocols specific for fish with cardiovascular disease are scarce. Several useful general formularies for fish are available to veterinarians.[10,29,46,52–54] There are also guides for emergency and critical care of fish.[55,56] In general, cardiovascular system–specific drugs or therapies are usually not characterized in fish formularies. The fish veterinarian needs to use sound clinical judgment based on the case history and clinical findings to choose and administer appropriate therapies.

Table 3 presents a suggested formulary for treating fish patients with suspected cardiac disease or in need of cardiac support. In addition to this, readers are encouraged to check current editions of exotic and zoo animal formularies that are readily available to clinical veterinarians and contain updated sections on fish therapeutics.[46,53,54] Proper treatment of a fish suspected of or proved to have cardiac disease may improve its quality of life and lifespan.

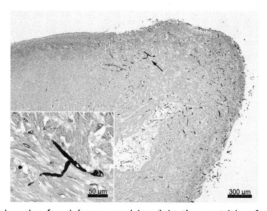

Fig. 13. Abundant invasive fungi (*arrow and inset*) in the ventricle of a juvenile Atlantic salmon (*Salmo salar*). Branched hyphae have nonparallel cell walls and poorly defined septae (probably *Saprolegnia* or a related species). Gomori methenamine silver stain.

Table 3
Suggested formulary for cardiac support and treatment of cardiac diseases in fish

Medication	Dose and Route	Indication/Comments	References
Antibiotics		For bacterial sepsis associated with cardiac infections, circulation failure, thrombosis	
Ceftazidime (Fortaz)	22 mg/kg IM, ICe q 72–96 hours for 3–5 treatments	Cephalosporin, good gram-negative spectrum	46
Enrofloxacin (Baytril)	5–10 mg/kg PO, IM, or ICe q 24–48 hours for up to 15 days 5 mg/kg PO or 0.1% (10 mg/10 g of feed) for 10–14 days 2.5–5 mg/L bath for 5 hours, repeated q 24 hours for 5–7 days	Gram-negative spectrum (eg, Aeromonas sp), injectable or oral form can be used for oral and bath treatments, 50%–75% water change recommended between bath treatments	46,78
Florfenicol (Nuflor)	20–30 mg/kg IM, ICe q 48 hours for 15 days	Labeled for treatment in food fish (eg, catfish, salmonids)	78
Metronidazole	50 mg/kg PO q 24 hours for 5 days 625 mg/100 g of feed for 5 days 0.2% (20 mg/20 g of feed) for 10 days 10 mg/L bath for 5–12 hours, repeated q 24 hours for 3 days 625 mg/10-gal bath for 6–8 hours	Anaerobes, also treats flagellates (eg, Uronema, Spironucleus)	2,46,78
Nitrofurazone	100 mg/L bath for 30 min 20 mg/L bath for 5 hours, repeated q 24 hours for 5–7 days 2–5 mg/L into tank water q 24 hours for 5–10 days	Caution: carcinogenic nitrofuran, use a water-soluble form, inactivated in bright light, 50%–75% water change recommended between bath treatments	46,78
Oxytetracycline	50–75 mg/kg PO q 24 hours 20 mg/kg PO q 24 hours for 10 days 10 mg/kg IM, ICe q 24 hours for 5–7 days 20–50 mg/L bath for 5–24 hours, repeated q 24 hours for 5–7 days	Binds to calcium in diet, bacterial resistance common, 50%–75% water change recommended between bath treatments	2,78
Trimethoprim/ sulfamethoxazole	50 mg/kg PO q 24 hours 30 mg/kg PO q 24 hours for 10–14 days 0.2% (20 mg/10 g of feed) for 10–14 days 20 mg/L bath for 5–12 hours, repeated q 24 hours for 5–7 days	50%–75% water change recommended between bath treatments	2,78

Antiparasitics

Larval and adult parasites can invade cardiac tissues, chambers, and vessels; parasite eggs can be virulent to cardiac tissues

Drug	Dosage	Comments	Ref
Fenbendazole	50 mg/kg PO q 7 days for three doses 0.2% (20 mg/10 g of feed) for 3 days, repeat in 14–21 days 2 mg/L into tank water q 7 days for 3 treatments	Nematodes (eg, Contracaecum larvae) in heart	2,46
Praziquantel	5 mg/kg PO q 24 hours for three treatments 50 mg/kg PO once 5 mg/kg ICe, repeat in 14–21 days 400 mg/100 g feed for 3–5 days 5–10-mg/L bath for 3–6 hours, repeat in 7 days	Cestode and trematode infestations; expensive; aerate water well; may cause lethargy, incoordination, loss of equilibrium	2,46
Antiarrhythmics			
Lidocaine	1–2 mg/kg IV as needed	Bolus for cardiac arrhythmias, used for ventricular tachycardia in mammals	10
Beta-blockers		β-adrenergic receptors in fish are similar to those in mammals	79
Atenolol		β_1 antagonist, may have no effect in certain fish; trout ventricular adrenoreceptors are exclusively β_2 type	80
Propranolol		Can block coronary vasodilatation, abolishes sympathetic influence on heart rate variability	79,81
Angiotensin-converting enzyme inhibitors		Used in mammals to decrease blood pressure, fluid retention, and afterload (by means of reduced vasoconstriction)	
Enalapril		No reported use in fish patients	
Vasodilators			
Nitroglycerin		Produced relaxation of coronary artery vascular rings in skates in vitro	82
Diuretics		Used in mammals to alleviate fluid retention secondary to congestive heart failure	

(continued on next page)

Table 3
(continued)

Medication	Dose and Route	Indication/Comments	References
Furosemide	2–5 mg/kg IM q 12–72 hours 2–3 mg/kg ICe, IM q 12 hours	Ascites or general edema (dropsy), questionable utility, fish lack a loop of Henle; lower range used in sharks	10,46
Mannitol	1–2 g/kg IV q 6 hours	Elevates plasma osmolality, osmotic diuresis	10
Cardiac support		May help in cases of suspected shock (eg, trauma, extreme stressors)	55,56
Atropine	2 mg/kg IM, ICe, IV 0.1 mg/kg IM, ICe, IV	Vascular stimulation, lower dose for organophosphate or hydrocarbon toxicity	10
Butorphanol (Torbugesic)	0.05–0.10 mg/kg IM 0.4 mg/kg IM (koi)	Analgesia, may cause mild sedation	46
Dexamethasone	1–2 mg/kg IM, ICe, IV 0.2–1.0 mg/kg PO	Glucocorticoid, cell stabilization in shock, higher dose for chlorine toxicity, anti-inflammatory effects at lower doses	28,46
Dextrose 5%	20–50 mL/kg ICe, IV	Reported for use as needed for dehydration in sharks	10
Doxapram	5 mg/kg ICe, IV	Respiratory depression	46
Epinephrine (1:1000)	0.2–0.5 mL IM, ICe, IV, IC	Cardiac arrest, rapid increase of coronary blood flow and dorsal aortic blood pressure (unrestrained salmon)	46,81
Heparin	200 U/kg ICe, IV q 4 hours	Disseminated intravascular coagulation in sharks, may help to prevent thrombosis during septicemia	10
Hydrocortisone	1–4 mg/kg IM, ICe 10 mg/L bath for 10–30 minutes	Shock, trauma, chronic stress	10,46
Hydrogen peroxide (3%)	0.25 mL/L bath for 10 minutes	Acute environmental hypoxia, oxygen may be more effective	46

Agent	Dose	Notes	References
Oxygen (100%)	2–4 mL/min per liter of water Inflate plastic bag containing one-third volume water	Acute hypoxia, useful for transport; helps to normalize coronary blood flow after hypoxia; avoid supersaturation of water with dissolved oxygen	46,81
Phenylephrine	0.15 mg/kg IV	α-Adrenergic agonist, vasoconstriction	10
Polyunsaturated n-3 fatty acids	High n-3/n-6 ratio feeds	Dietary sources, fish oil; may aid resistance of hypoxia-induced stress effects on heart tissue	27,77
Prednisolone	1 mg/kg IV, ICe, IM	Shock support in sharks	10
Salt (sodium chloride)	30–35 g/L dip for 4–5 minutes 10–30 g/L dip for up to 30 minutes 1–5 g/L added to tank water indefinitely	Supportive care for stressed freshwater fish; artificial sea salts preferable, can use non-ionized table or rock salts; dips treat some freshwater fish ectoparasites	46
Anesthetic agents			
Ketamine/medetomidine	1–2 mg/kg ketamine + 0.05–0.10 mg/kg medetomidine IM 6 mg/kg ketamine + 0.06 mg/kg medetomidine IM 4 mg/kg ketamine + 0.4 mg/kg medetomidine IM	Ketamine is an FDA-controlled drug, reverse medetomidine portion with atipamezole (0.2–0.3 mg/kg IM), bradycardia and respiratory depression possible, wide interspecies variations in dose and response	46,83,84
Propofol	2.5–6.5 mg/kg IV to effect	Requires venous access, bradycardia and respiratory depression possible, lower dose: stable cardiorespiratory parameters in spotted bamboo sharks, higher dose: light plane of anesthesia in sturgeon	83,85
Tricaine methanesulfonate (MS 222, Finquel)	8–30 mg/L or 15–50-mg/L bath for sedation 50–100 mg/L bath for induction 50–60 mg/L for maintenance 100–200 mg/L bath, 10 minutes longer than respiratory arrest for euthanasia	Adjustable levels of anesthesia possible; FDA-approved in food fish; stock solution 10 g/L, buffered with sodium bicarbonate at 10 g/L; shelf life increased with light protection, refrigeration, or freezing	2,45,46

Abbreviations: FDA, Federal Drug Administration; IC, intracardiac; ICe, intracoelomically; IM, intramuscularly; IV, intravenously; PO, orally; q, every.

SUMMARY

Published reports of cardiovascular disease in companion and display fish are uncommon, perhaps because of a paucity of consistent postmortem examinations and clinical studies in client-owned or aquarium fish. Cardiovascular system lesions clearly occur in many fish species, however, as evidenced by finfish aquaculture research and general fish research bodies of literature.

Undoubtedly, veterinarians can successfully draw from methodologies used for nonaquatic pets to evaluate the cardiovascular system of pet or display fish. Systematic diagnostic testing followed by application of logical treatment for identified primary or secondary cardiac problems may prolong the lifespan of an affected fish patient. It is hoped that this summary of current knowledge aids in the diagnosis and treatment of fish cardiovascular diseases and stimulates subsequent publication of new findings.

ACKNOWLEDGMENTS

The authors thank Dr. Greg Lewbart and Shane Christian at the College of Veterinary Medicine at North Carolina State University for their contributions regarding koi heart lesions and Dr. Alan Klide at the School of Veterinary Medicine at the University of Pennsylvania for his images of cardiac monitoring in fish. Special gratitude is extended to Jadzia and Andrzej Jazac for their invaluable assistance to Dr. Sherrill.

REFERENCES

1. Graham JB, Dickson KA. Anatomical and physiological specializations for endothermy. In: Block BA, Stevens ED, editors. Tuna: physiological ecology and evolution. San Diego (CA): Academic Press; 2001. p. 121–60.
2. Whitaker BR. Common disorders of marine fish. In: Rosenthal K, editor. Practical exotic animal medicine. Trenton (NJ): Veterinary Learning Systems Co., Inc.; 1997. p. 230–6.
3. Tota B. Myoarchitecture and vascularization of the elasmobranch heart ventricle. In: Hamlett WC, Tota B, editors. Evolutionary and contemporary biology of elasmobranchs. J Exp Zool 1989;(Suppl 2):1–196.
4. Randall DJ. The circulatory system. In: Hoar WS, Randall DJ, editors, Fish physiology: the nervous system, circulation, and respiration, vol. 4. London: Academic Press; 1970. p. 133–72.
5. Fange R. Fish blood cells. Part B. In: Hoar WS, Randall DJ, Farrell AP, editors. Fish physiology, vol. 12. Part B. San Diego (CA): Academic Press; 1992. p. 1–54.
6. Nakamura H, Shimozawa A. Phagocytotic cells in the fish heart. Arch Histol Cytol 1994;57(4):415–25.
7. Thorson TB. The partitioning of body water in Osteichthyes: phylogenetic and ecological implications in aquatic vertebrates. Biol Bull 1961;120:238–54.
8. Satchell GH. Physiology and form of fish circulation. New York: Cambridge University Press; 1991.
9. DeVries AL, Eastman JT. Physiology and ecology of Notothenioid fishes of the Ross Sea. J Royal Society of New Zealand 1981;11(4):329–40.
10. Stoskopf MK. Fish medicine. Philadelphia: W.B. Saunders; 1993.
11. Vogel WOP. The caudal heart of fishes: not a lymph heart. Acta Anat 1985;121: 41–5.

12. Olsen KR, Farrell AP. The cardiovascular system. In: Evans DH, Claiborne JB, editors. The physiology of fishes. 3rd edition. Boca Raton (FL): CRC Press; 2006. p. 119–42.

13. Hewson W, Hunter W. An account of the lymphatic system in amphibious animals. By Mr. William Hewson, Lecturer in Anatomy: In a Letter to William Hunter, M.D.F.R.S. and by Him Communicated to the Society, vol. 59. Philosophical transactions (1683–1775);1769. p. 198–203.

14. Harder W. The digestive tract. In: Schwizerbart'sche S, editor. Anatomy of fishes 1975. p. 128–87.

15. Küchler AM, Gjini E, Peterson-Maduro J, et al. Development of the zebrafish lymphatic system requires VEGFC signaling. Curr Biol 2006;16(12):1244–8.

16. Santer RM. Morphology and innervation of the fish heart. Adv Anat Embryol Cell Biol 1985;89:1–99.

17. Sanchez-Quintana D, Garcia-Martinez V, Climent V, et al. Morphological analysis of the fish heart ventricle: myocardial and connective tissue architecture in teleost species. Ann Anat 1995;177:267–74.

18. Icardo JM, Imbrogno S, Gattuso A, et al. The heart of Sparus auratus: a reappraisal of cardiac functional morphology in teleosts. J Exp Zool 2005;303A(8): 665–75.

19. Coleman FC. Morphological and physiological consequences of parasites encysted in the bulbus arteriosus of an estuarine fish, the Sheepshead Minnow, Cyprinodon variegatus. J Parasitol 1993;79(2):247–54.

20. Shiels HA, Calaghan SC, White E. The cellular basis for enhanced volume-modulated cardiac output in fish hearts. J Gen Physiol 2006;128(1):37–44.

21. Altimiras J, Aissaoui A, Tort L. Is the short-term modulation of heart rate in teleost fish physiologically significant? Assessment by spectral analysis techniques. Braz J Med Biol Res 1995;28:1197–206.

22. Mott JC. The cardiovascular system. In: Brown ME, editor. The physiology of fishes, vol. 1. New York: Academic Press; 1957. p. 81–105.

23. Haverinen J, Vornanen M. Temperature acclimation modifies sinoatrial pacemaker mechanism of the rainbow trout heart. Am J Physiol Regul Integr Comp Physiol 2007;292(2):1023–32.

24. Gamperl KA, Farrell AP. Cardiac plasticity in fishes: environmental influences and intraspecific differences. J Exp Biol 2004;207:2539–50.

25. Beleau MH. Evaluating water problems. Vet Clin North Am Small Anim Pract 1988; 18:317–30.

26. Leknes IL. Ultrastructural and ultrahistochemical studies of post-mortem changes and effects of hypoxia in the bony fish heart. J Submicrosc Cytol Pathol 1985; 17(2):223–8.

27. Agnisola C, McKenzie DJ, Taylor EW, et al. Cardiac performance in relation to oxygen supply varies with dietary lipid composition in sturgeon. Am J Physiol 1996;271:417–25.

28. Citino SB. Basic ornamental fish medicine. In: Kirk RW, Bonagura JD, editors. Current veterinary therapy X. Philadelphia: W.B. Saunders; 1989. p. 703–21.

29. Lewbart GA. Medical management of disorders of freshwater tropical fish. In: Rosenthal K, editor. Practical exotic animal medicine. Trenton (NJ): Veterinary Learning Systems Co., Inc; 1997. p. 250–7.

30. Harms CA. Fish. In: Fowler ME, Miller RE, editors. Zoo and wild animal medicine: current therapy 4. Philadelphia: W.B. Saunders; 1999. p. 158–63.

31. Noga EJ. Fish disease: diagnosis and treatment. Ames (IA): Iowa State University Press; 2000.

32. Weber ES, Innis C. Piscine patients: basic diagnostics. Compend Contin Educ Vet 2007;29(5):276–7, 280, 282–6 [quiz: 286, 288].
33. Reimschuessel R. Necropsy techniques in aquarium fish. In: Bonagura JD, editor. Kirk's current veterinary therapy XII: small animal practice. Philadelphia: W.B. Saunders; 1995. p. 1198–203.
34. McLoughlin MF, Graham DA. Alphavirus infections in salmonids—a review. J Fish Dis 2007;30(9):511–31.
35. Kongtorp RT, Halse M, Taksdal T, et al. Longitudinal study of a natural outbreak of heart and skeletal muscle inflammation in Atlantic salmon, Salmo salar. J Fish Dis 2006;29(4):233–44.
36. Noga EJ. Biopsy and rapid postmortem techniques for diagnosing diseases of fish. Vet Clin North Am Small Anim Pract 1998;18(2):401–26.
37. Sande RD, Poppe TT. Diagnostic ultrasound examination and echocardiography in Atlantic salmon (Salmo salar). Vet Radiol Ultrasound 1995;36(6):551–8.
38. Lai NC, Dalton N, Lai YY, et al. A comparative echocardiographic assessment of ventricular function in five species of sharks. Comp Biochem Physiol A Mol Integr Physiol 2004;137(3):505–21.
39. Van der Linden A, Verhoye M, Poertner HO, et al. The strengths of in vivo magnetic resonance imaging (MRI) to study environmental adaptational physiology in fish. MAGMA 2004;17(3–6):236–48.
40. Murray MJ. Endoscopy in fish. In: Murray MJ, Schildger B, Taylor M, editors. Endoscopy in birds, reptiles, amphibians and fish. Tuttlingen (Germany): Endo-Press. p. 59–75.
41. Boone S, Hernandez-Divers SJ, et al. Comparison between celioscopy and coeliotomy for live biopsy in channel catfish (Ictalurus punctatus). J Am Vet Med Assoc, in press.
42. Korsmeyer KE, Chin Lai N, Shadwick RE, et al. Oxygen transport and cardiovascular responses to exercise in the yellowfin tuna (Thunnus albacares). J Exp Biol 1997;200:1987–97.
43. Cooper R, Krum H, Tzinas G, et al. A preliminary study of clinical techniques utilized with bluefin tuna (Thunnus thynnus): a comparison of some captive and wild caught blood parameters. Proceedings of the 25th International Association of Aquatic Animal Medicine Conference. Vallejo (CA); 1994. p. 26–35.
44. Tebecis AK. A study of electrograms recorded from the conus arteriosus of an elasmobranch heart. Aust J Biol Sci 1967;20:843–6.
45. American Veterinary Medical Association (AVMA) guidelines on euthanasia. Avaliable at: http://www.avma.org/issues/animal_welfare/euthanasia.pdf. Accessed June 2007.
46. Carpenter JW. Exotic animal formulary: fish. Philadelphia: Elsevier; 2005. p. 5–29.
47. Ferguson HW. Systemic pathology of fish. 2nd edition. Ames (IA): Iowa State University Press; 2006.
48. Roberts RJ. Fish pathology. 3rd edition. London: Bailliere Tindall; 2001.
49. Reite OB. The rodlet cells of teleostean fish: their potential role in host defence in relation to the role of mast cells/eosinophilic granule cells. Fish Shellfish Immunol 2005;19(3):253–67.
50. Brown LA. Anesthesia in fish. Vet Clin North Am Small Anim Pract 1988;18:291–316.
51. Stoskofp MK. Anesthesia of pet fishes. In: Bonagura JD, editor. Kirk's current veterinary therapy XII: small animal practice. Philadelphia: W.B. Saunders; 1995. p. 1365–9.
52. Harms CA. Anesthesia in fish. In: Fowler ME, Miller RE, editors. Zoo and wild animal medicine. 5th edition. Philadelphia: W.B. Saunders; 2003. p. 2–20.

53. Stoskofp MK. Fish pharmacotherapeutics. In: Fowler ME, Miller RE, editors. Zoo and wild animal medicine: current therapy 4. Philadelphia: W.B. Saunders; 1999. p. 182–9.
54. Whitaker BR. Preventive medicine programs for fish. In: Fowler ME, Miller RE, editors. Zoo and wild animal medicine: current therapy 4. Philadelphia: W.B. Saunders; 1999. p. 163–81.
55. Lewbart GA. Emergency and critical care of fish. Vet Clin North Am Exot Anim Pract 1998;1:233–49.
56. Hadfield C, Whitaker B, Clayton L. Emergency and critical care of fish. Vet Clin North Am Exot Anim Pract 2007;10(2):647–75.
57. Rowley HM, Doherty CE, McLoughlin MF, et al. Isolation of salmon pancreas disease virus (SPDV) from farmed Atlantic salmon, *Salmo salar* L., in Scotland. J Fish Dis 1998;21(6):469–71.
58. Kongtorp RT, Taksdal T, Lyngoy A. Pathology of heart and skeletal muscle inflammation (HSMI) in farmed Atlantic salmon *Salmo salar*. Dis Aquat Organ 2004; 59(3):217–24.
59. Lumsden JS, Morrison B, Yason C, et al. Mortality event in freshwater drum *Aplodinotus grunniens* from Lake Ontario, Canada, associated with viral haemorrhagic septicemia virus, type IV. Dis Aquat Organ 2007;76(2):99–111.
60. Hayakawa Y, Harada T, Hatai K, et al. Histopathology of BKD (bacterial kidney disease) occurred in sea-cultured coho salmon (*Oncorhynchus kisutch*). Fish Pathol 1989;24:17–21.
61. Stine CB, Baya AM, Salierno JD, et al. Mycobacterial infection in laboratory-maintained Atlantic menhaden (*Brevoortia tyrannus*). J Aquat Anim Health 2005;17: 380–5.
62. Chen SC, Lee JL, Lai CC, et al. Nocardiosis in sea bass, *Lateolabrax japonicus*, in Taiwan. J Fish Dis 2000;23(5):299–307.
63. Marty GD, Freiberg EF, Meyers TR, et al. Viral hemorrhagic septicemia virus, *Ichthyophonus hoferi*, and other causes of morbidity in Pacific herring *Clupea pallasi* spawning in Prince William Sound, Alaska. Dis Aquat Org 1998;32(1): 15–40.
64. Dick TA. The atrium of the fish heart as a site for *Contracaecum sp.* larvae. J Wildl Dis 1987;23(2):328–30.
65. Belem AMG, Pote LM. Portals of entry and systemic localization of proliferative gill disease organisms in channel catfish *Ictalurus punctatus*. Dis Aquat Org 2001;48(1):37–42.
66. Masoumian M, Baska F, Malnar K. Description of *Myxobolus bulbocordis sp.* nov. (Myxosporea: Myxobolidae) from the heart of *Barbus sharpeyi* (Guenther) and histopathological changes produced by the parasite. J Fish Dis 1996;19(1): 15–21.
67. Toerud B, Taksdal T, Dale OB, et al. Myocardial glycogen storage disease in farmed rainbow trout, *Oncorhynchus mykiss* (Walbaum). J Fish Dis 2006;29(9): 535–40.
68. Poppe TT, Taksdal T. Ventricular hypoplasia in farmed Atlantic salmon *Salmo salar*. Dis Aquat Org 2000;42(1):35–40.
69. Poppe TT, Johansen R, Torud B. Cardiac abnormality with associated hernia in farmed rainbow trout *Oncorhynchus mykiss*. Dis Aquat Org 2002;50(2):153–5.
70. Farrell AP, Saunders RL, Freeman HC, et al. Arteriosclerosis in Atlantic salmon. Effects of dietary cholesterol and maturation. Arteriosclerosis 1986;6(4):453–61.
71. Heidel JR, LaPatra SE, Giles J. Mineralization of the bulbus arteriosus in adult rainbow trout *Oncorhynchus mykiss*. J Vet Diagn Invest 1997;9(2):213–6.

72. Smith MP, Dombkowski RA, Wincko JT, et al. Effect of pH on trout blood vessels and gill vascular resistance. J Exp Biol 2006;209(13):2586–94.

73. Johansen R, Poppe T. Pericarditis and myocarditis in farmed Atlantic halibut *Hippoglossus hippoglossus*. Dis Aquat Org 2002;49(1):77–81.

74. Brocklebank J, Raverty S. Sudden mortality caused by cardiac deformities following seining of preharvest farmed Atlantic salmon (*Salmo salar*) and by cardiomyopathy of postintraperitoneally vaccinated Atlantic salmon parr in British Columbia. Can Vet J 2002;43(2):129–30.

75. Couch JA. Invading and metastasizing cardiac hemangioendothelial neoplasms in a cohort of the fish *Rivulus marmoratus*: unusually high prevalence, histopathology, and possible etiologies. Cancer Res 1995;55:2438–47.

76. Shields RP, Popp JA. Intracardial mesotheliomas and a gastric papilloma in a giant grouper, *Epinephelus itajara*. Vet Pathol 1979;16(2):191–8.

77. Bell JG, McVicar AH, Park MT, et al. High dietary linoleic acid affects the fatty acid compositions of individual phospholipids from tissues of Atlantic salmon (*Salmo salar*): association with stress susceptibility and cardiac lesion. J Nutr 1991; 121(8):1163–72.

78. Lewbart GA. CVT update: antibiotic treatment of aquarium fish. In: Bonagura JD, editor. Kirk's current veterinary therapy XIII: small animal practice. Philadelphia: W.B. Saunders; 2000. p. 1196–8.

79. Owen SF, Giltrow E, Huggett DB, et al. Comparative physiology, pharmacology and toxicology of beta-blockers: mammals versus fish. Aquat Toxicol 2007; 82(3):145–62.

80. Gamperl AK, Wilkinson M, Boutilier RG. Beta-adrenoreceptors in the trout (*Oncorhynchus mykiss*) heart: characterization, quantification, and effects of repeated catecholamine exposure. Gen Comp Endocrinol 1994;95:259–72.

81. Axelsson M, Farrell AP. Coronary blood flow in vivo in the coho salmon (*Oncorhynchus-kisutch*). Am J Physiol 1993;264(5):963–71.

82. Farrell AP, Davie PS. Coronary vascular reactivity in the skate Raja nasuta. Comp Biochem Physiol C, Pharmacol Toxicol Endocrinol 1991;99(3):555–60.

83. Fleming GJ, Heard DJ, Francis-Floyd RF, et al. Evaluation of propofol and medetomidine-ketamine for short-term immobilization of Gulf of Mexico sturgeon (Acipenser oxyrinchus de soti). J Zoo Wildl Med 2003;34(2):153–8.

84. Williams TD, Rollins M, Block BA. Intramuscular anesthesia of bonito and Pacific mackerel with ketamine and medetomidine and reversal of anesthesia with atipamezole. J Am Vet Med Assoc 2004;225(3):417–21.

85. Miller SM, Mitchell MA, Heatley JJ, et al. Clinical and cardiorespiratory effects of propofol in the spotted bamboo shark (*Chylloscyllium Plagiosum*). J Zoo Wildl Med 2005;36(4):673–6.

Cardiovascular Physiology and Diseases of Amphibians

Kathleen M. Heinz-Taheny, DVM, PhD, DACVP

KEYWORDS

- Cardiovascular • Amphibian • Anuran
- Salamander • Caecilian • *Xenopus*

The class Amphibia includes three orders of amphibians: the anurans (frogs and toads), urodeles (salamanders, axolotls, and newts), and caecilians. The diversity of lifestyles across these three orders has accompanying differences in the cardiovascular anatomy and physiology allowing for adaptations to aquatic or terrestrial habitats, pulmonic or gill respiration, hibernation, and body elongation (in the caecilian). This article provides a review of amphibian cardiovascular anatomy and physiology with discussion of unique species adaptations. In addition, amphibians as cardiovascular animal models and commonly encountered natural diseases are covered.

ANATOMY AND PHYSIOLOGY

Blood flow through the amphibian heart follows a complicated pathway to prevent the mixing of oxygenated and deoxygenated blood in the three-chambered heart (**Fig. 1**). Less oxygenated blood returning to the heart through the venous system flows through the anterior and posterior caval veins, the sinus venosus, and empties into the right atrium. Blood within the venous system entering the heart contains oxygen and is low in carbon dioxide based on both cutaneous and buccal respiration. The left atrium receives blood oxygenated via the lungs and the skin. Blood from both atria empties into the single ventricle. In species possessing an interatrial septum, contraction of the atrial septum and the dorsal aspect of the atria decreases the atrial capacity and increases the capacity of the sinus venosus. The decreased atrial capacity forces blood into the ventricle while the increased capacity in the sinus venosus draws blood from the venous system consisting of the three caval veins.[1]

The single ventricle reduces the mixing of oxygenated and deoxygenated blood by extensive trabeculation of the ventricular wall and by a complicated system of biphasic contractions.[1,2] Mixing of blood from the left and right atria is also prevented by the ventricular portion of the atrial septum. The volume of the single ventricle is less

Lilly Research Laboratories, Eli Lilly and Co., 355 E. Merrill Street, Indianapolis IN 46225, USA
E-mail address: heinztahenykm@lilly.com (K.M. Heinz-Taheny).

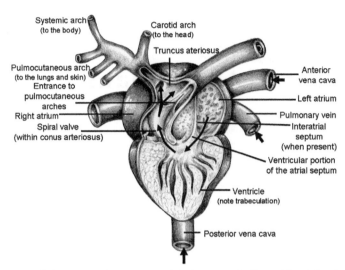

Fig. 1. Anatomy of the anuran heart. Large block arrows indicate blood flowing into the heart. Thin black arrows indicate flow of oxygenated blood. (*Courtesy of* Frank Taheny.)

than both atria and therefore the ventricle cannot hold all of the blood from both atria at one time.[1] Despite the lack of an interventricular septum in most amphibians, the flow of oxygenated and deoxygenated blood is differentially directed by multiple factors including volume and position of the blood within the ventricle, alterations in ventricular contractions, arterial branching patterns, and pressure differences in the pulmonary and systemic vasculature.[3] Separation of blood into the three arches (pulmocutaneous, systemic, and carotid) is accomplished by the hinge-like movement of the spiral valve in the conus arteriosus, a transition between the heart and the vascular system. Pressure exerted from the pulmocutaneous chamber moves the spiral valve upward to separate the pulmocutaneous chamber from the systemocarotid chamber.[1,4,5] In the first phase of ventricular systole, blood on the right side of the ventricle (less oxygenated) moves into the pulmocutaneous arch. Deoxygenated blood flows from the ventricle into the pulmocutaneous arteries and then to the lungs and skin for gas exchange. In the second phase of ventricular systole, blood from the left side of the ventricle (oxygenated) moves into the systemic and carotid arches aided by alignment of these arches with the ventricle and pressure within the pulmocutaneous arch. During this second phase of ventricular systole, there is the potential for a small amount of mixing of blood within the ventricle as blood makes its way into the systemocarotid vasculature. Contraction of the conus arteriosus forces blood simultaneously through both these vessels.[1] The carotid arch supplies the head. The systemic arch supplies the body.

The degree of mixing of oxygenated and deoxygenated blood in the amphibian heart has been determined based on an extensive experiment in the heart of *Xenopus laevis*.[6] In this model, blood from the right atrium remains on the right side of the ventricle and marginal quantities of blood from the right atrium reach the left side of the ventricle. However, a considerable portion of the blood from the left atrium reaches the right half of the ventricle. Most of the blood from the right atrium is sent to the pulmocutaneous arches and most of the blood from the left atrium is sent to the carotid and systemic arches. With each heartbeat, more blood flows through the pulmocutaneous arches than the carotid and systemic arches combined. Blood flow through the pulmonary circulation is substantially greater than the flow through the body circulation and resistance in the pulmocutaneous arch is consistently lower than the carotid or systemic arches owing to reduced pressure in the pulmocutaneous system. However, pressures in the carotid and systemic arches are similar.

ANATOMIC DIFFERENCES

Although the general morphology of the heart is similar across the three orders of amphibians, there are slight differences. Typically, the right atrium is larger than the left atrium in most salamanders and anurans but the atria are of equal size in a few anurans, most notably in *X laevis*. In contrast, the right atrium in caecilians is smaller than the left.[7] The interatrial septum is complete in anurans and in the salamander genus *Siren*. The septum is fenestrated in caecilians and other salamanders.[8,9] A comparison of three urodeles demonstrates alterations in cardiac anatomy with different habitats. *Siren lacertina,* a primarily pulmonic salamander possesses a complete interatrial septum, whereas two nonpulmonary respiring species, *Necturus maculosus* that respire by external gills and *Cryptobranchus alleganiensis* that rely on cutaneous respiration, both have fenestrated interatrial septa.[9,10] The interatrial septum of plethodontid salamanders is membranous, lacks fenestration, and has a sinoatrial valve that regulates blood flow between atria. This valve likely occurs because of the lack of a pulmonary vein in these lungless salamanders. Further, the membranous interatrial septum may allow the sinoatrial opening to supply blood to both atria and prevent left-sided stagnation because of the lack of a pulmonary vein.[9]

While the ventricle in most anurans and caecilians is a single chamber, salamanders have a sinoventricular fold that is absent in anurans and caecilians.[7] Two genera of salamanders take it a step further with a partially septate ventricular division. The ventricle is divided in *Siren* spp and *Necturus* spp salamanders by an incomplete interventricular septum created by the muscular trabeculae of the ventricular wall and divides the ventricle into a smaller left and larger right chamber assisting in segregation of the oxygenated and deoxygenated blood.[8,11,12] Separation of the blood is likely complete in these two genera.[8,11] In addition, *Necturus* spp and *Siren intermedia* also possess an intraventricular septum within the right ventricular chamber.[11,12]

In salamanders, the sinus venosus is not divided except in the *Siren* in which there is an incomplete longitudinal septum separating the sinus venosus into major right and minor left chambers.[8] In anurans, a constriction of the inner wall divides the sinus venosus into right and left sides. In caecilians, indentations of the wall of the sinus or a pair of transverse valves divide the sinus venosus.[7] The conus arteriosus in some plethodontid salamander species lacks the spiral valve.[13] Caecilian studies have not been conducted on circulation but based on anatomic characteristics, it is probable that ventricular mixing of oxygenated and deoxygenated blood occurs, although the extensive ventricular trabeculation may partially separate oxygenated and deoxygenated blood. As expected for an elongated animal, the truncus arteriosus is also elongated in the caecilian but shortened in anurans and salamanders.[7]

BEHAVIORAL INFLUENCE ON BLOOD FLOW

Blood volume and speed through the heart and vasculature is variable depending on the lifestyle of the amphibian (terrestrial versus aquatic) and physiologic state (active versus hibernating). Terrestrial species of frogs have larger hearts than aquatic species and this may reflect increased work against gravity in these species or an increased aerobic demand of land habitation.[14,15] Ventricular weights were comparably greater in the terrestrial species than aquatic and semi-aquatic species.[15]

Hibernating aquatic amphibians adjust their cardiovascular system to conserve blood flow to oxygen-sensitive organs such as the brain, heart, and kidney resulting in hypoperfusion of hypoxia-tolerant tissues such as inactive skeletal muscle during hibernation. In bullfrogs (*Rana catesbiana*), perfusion of lungs and skin by pulmocutaneous blood flow redistribute based on the environmental type. Lung perfusion, which approached 80% in control conditions, increased during water hypoxia but was reduced when frogs inspired hypoxic air. Skin perfusion was reduced during aquatic hypoxia to allow increased perfusion of the lung and increased when inspiring oxygen-poor air. These findings may reflect blood redirection to areas of gas exchange or represent a mechanism to prevent oxygen loss at sites of lowered oxygen tension. This ability to divert pulmocutaneous blood flow away from the lungs and to the skin during conditions of low pulmonary Po_2 also may serve to alleviate hypoxic conditions during diving. The ventrum of amphibians is the area of skin most highly perfused by the pulmocutaneous artery making this region the most important location of gas and ion exchange.[16]

VASCULATURE

The number of aortic arches that persist into adulthood varies across the three orders with most amphibians lacking the first two arches and only some salamanders containing the full set. Branching from the truncus arteriosus, the carotid arch (visceral arch III) delivers blood to the head; the systemic arch (visceral arch IV) delivers blood to the body with some flow to the head excluding the pharynx, lungs, and variable distribution to the skin; and the pulmonary arch (visceral arch VI) supplies the lungs, the walls of the pharynx, and cutaneous branches (**Fig. 2**). The third arch (visceral arch V) is present in some salamander species but adult anurans lack this arch. In caecilians, only two arches are found: the pulmonary and the fused systemic and carotid.[7]

Hepatic-Portal System

The ventral abdominal vein is formed by the merging of pelvic veins in anurans and also includes the union of the median cloacal and posterior vesicle veins from the

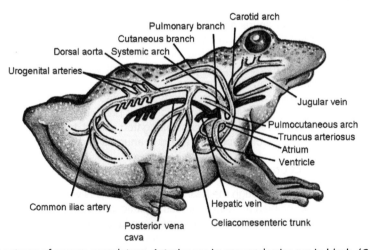

Fig. 2. Anatomy of anuran vasculature. Arteries are in gray and veins are in black. (*Courtesy of* Frank Taheny.)

cloaca and bladder respectively in the salamander. The ventral abdominal vein courses along the ventral midline through the liver to the postcaval vein. Near the liver, the vein receives vesicle veins from the gall bladder and portal vein with branches from the stomach and intestines.[7] Drug administration of hepatically metabolized compounds in the caudal half of the amphibian should be avoided because the pharmacokinetics of the drug could be significantly or unexpectedly affected.

Renal-Portal System

The venous system of the hindlimbs of the amphibian body fuses into the paired Jacobson's veins, which pass anteriorly on the dorsolateral surface of the kidney. The oviductal vein also empties into Jacobson's veins, which terminate into the postcaval vein.[7] Drug administration of renally metabolized or excreted compounds in the caudal half of the amphibian should be avoided because the pharmacokinetics of the drug could be significantly affected. Because of this pattern of blood flow, known nephrotic drugs should not be administered in the caudal half of an amphibian.

LYMPHATICS

The lymphatic system is an extensive network of endothelial-lined vessels and dilated sinuses located within the musculature, mesentery, and subcutaneous tissue. Anurans have large subcutaneous lymph sinuses not found in the other orders of amphibians. The anuran subcutis is entirely composed of lymph sacs. Lymph is composed of plasma and leukocytes but a comparison of plasma and lymph has not been well documented.[17] Intestinal lymphatics also collect fat.[7]

Anatomy

Paired lymph hearts, located dorsally in the subcutaneous tissue, pump lymph independently of cardiac rate. The anterior pair is located on the dorsal surface of the transverse processes of the third vertebrae just beneath the scapula. The posterior hearts, which may be a single pair or up to five pairs, are located laterally, on each side of the urostyle.[18,19] The superficial location allows visualization of their pulsation through the skin. Lymph hearts do not beat synchronously but rhythmically, averaging about 50 to 60 beats per minute.[18] Tissue fluid composed of blood and water absorbed through the skin diffuses into subcutaneous lymph capillaries that move into larger lymph vessels and into lymph spaces. The lymph hearts and skeletal muscle contraction drive this movement and the passage of lymph into communicating veins.[18,20] The anterior hearts drain fluid into the anterior vertebral veins and the posterior into the renal portal system.[19] There is a central lymph heart associated with the truncus arteriosus that receives lymph from the head and neck and empties into the lingual vein.[7]

Movement of lymph hearts can be stopped by administration of curare, which prevents the return of lymph to the blood and results in dilation of lymph sacs and edema. Experimentally, paralysis of the lymph hearts in frogs remaining in an aquatic environment resulted in body weight gains of 10% to 30% in 6 hours.[18]

Lymph valves maintain unidirectional lymph flow and have associated musculature allowing the valves to tense and tighten the valve, aiding in maintaining pressure within the circuit.[18,21] Movement of lymph is also enhanced by physical activity of the animal and experimental severance of muscle groups resulted in lymph pooling in dependent lymph sacs.[19,20]

Species and Lifestyle Anatomic Differences

Caecilians possess the most number of lymph hearts with greater than 200, salamanders have about 10 to 20, and anurans have few lymph hearts.[7]

In anurans, interspecific variability in lymph sac size is correlated with habitat use.[19] As the anuran became more terrestrial, the lymph sacs become reduced in size. Accordingly, aquatic species have the largest lymph sacs. Aquatic species may require relatively large lymph sacs to move additional cutaneously absorbed water from their habitat, whereas terrestrial species have a lower water burden because they rarely submerge in water. In addition, fine septa that separate lymph spaces are most extensive in aquatic anurans. These spaces store absorbed water. Excess water is excreted by the posterior lymph hearts by moving water from these lymph spaces into the renal portal vein where it is voided through the kidneys.[19]

Clinical Consequences

Lymph samples may be obtained from a large prominent pair of lymph sacs located dorsally along the sides of the urostyle in terrestrial anurans.[17] The large volume of lymph moved and the quickness by which the lymph hearts circulate lymph may make sampling lymph difficult in a healthy amphibian. Accumulation of large amounts of lymph in sacs indicates illness (**Fig. 3**). Hydrated amphibians may direct fluid absorbed cutaneously into the lymphatics and bypass arterial blood, which may bear implications on the absorption and distribution of cutaneously administered pharmaceuticals.[17,22]

CARDIOVASCULAR DISEASES: INFECTIOUS ETIOLOGIES

Involvement of the heart in cases of bacterial septicemia is relatively rare despite the high incidence of gram-negative septicemias. No bacterial infections are known that specifically target the amphibian heart. Generalized ("hydrops") or localized edema is a common, nonspecific presentation for multiple untoward conditions in amphibians including vascular alterations (**Fig. 4**). Infectious agents causing hydrops include many

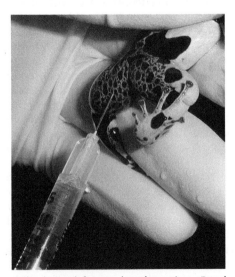

Fig. 3. Lymph fluid is easily drained from a lymph sac in a *Dendrobates tinctorius* with hydrops. (*Courtesy of* the National Aquarium in Baltimore, MD.)

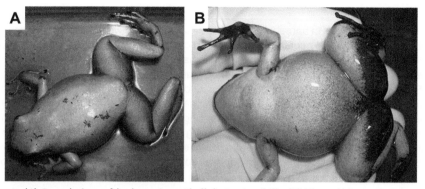

Fig. 4. (*A*) Dorsal view of hydrops in a *Phyllobates terribilis.* (*B*) Ventral view of the same animal. (*Courtesy of* the National Aquarium in Baltimore, MD.)

gram-negative and some gram-positive bacteria. Although the list is exhaustive, notable agents include *Aeromonas hydrophila, Flavobacterium spp,* and *Chlamydophila Spp.*

Mycobacterium Spp

Systemic mycobacterial infections are commonly encountered in amphibians. *Mycobacterium marinum* is ubiquitous in aquatic environments and responsible for zoonotic infections causing skin lesions termed "aquarist's nodules," "fish tank granulomas," or "swimming pool granulomas." Disseminated human infection occurs rarely in immunosuppressed individuals.[23] *Mycobacterium fortuitum, Mycobacterium chelonae, M marinum, Mycobacterium liflandii, Mycobacterium thamnopheos,* and *Mycobacterium xenopi* are known to infect amphibians.[24,25] The author has diagnosed and managed multiple outbreaks of mycobacterial infections in laboratory-reared *X laevis.* Elimination of this bacterium from aquatic systems is challenging and recurrence is frequent following repopulation. Diagnosis by acid-fast staining is best accomplished using Fite's acid-fast technique (instead of Ziehl-Neelsen) in amphibian species (**Fig. 5**).

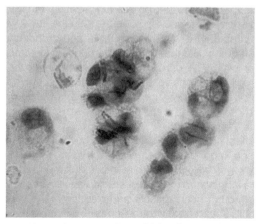

Fig. 5. Aspirate of a granuloma demonstrating acid-fast bacteria consistent with *Mycobacterium* spp within macrophages. (*Courtesy of* the National Aquarium in Baltimore, MD.)

Chlamydophila Spp

Chlamydial infections in anurans occur in both wild and captive populations. *Chlamydophila* spp are gram-negative, obligate intracellular cocci.[26] The most frequently isolated species causing disease in amphibians are *Chlamydophila psittaci* and *Chlamydophila pneumoniae,* although a recent survey of chlamydial infections in frogs in Switzerland also identified *Chlamydia suis* and *Chlamydophila abortus,* although no lesions were associated with infection.[26,27] African clawed frogs (*X laevis*) infected with *Chlamydophila* spp often develop a necrotizing and granulomatous epicarditis and myocarditis.[28] A captive Blue Mountain tree frog *(Litoria citropa)* developed a nonsuppurative chronic epicarditis with histologically evident intracellular, intracytoplasmic organisms consistent with *Chlamydophila* spp infection and determined to be *C pneumoniae.*[26]

Systemic Fungi

Systemic fungal infections in amphibians periodically result in cardiac granuloma formation and include candidiasis, zygomycosis, geotrichosis, chromomycosis, and phaehyphomycosis, among other species.[29,30]

Iridovirus

The Iridoviridae family includes multiple viruses that infect amphibians. These highly virulent viruses cause systemic disease and tadpoles are the most susceptible to infection, dying abruptly with no clinical signs.[31] Most notable are two from the genus *Ranavirus:* frog virus 3 and tadpole edema virus. Amphibians develop a generalized viremia and multiple organ systems may be affected. Cardiac lesions noted in tiger salamanders (*Ambystoma tigrinum*) included intracytoplasmic myocyte viral inclusions, pyknotic myocytes, and myocardial necrosis sometimes resulting in heart failure.[32,33] The isolated iridovirus was Regina ranavirus.[33]

Parasites

Trematode larvae of various species frequently encyst in cardiac muscle and may cause clinical infection. The strigeoid metacercaria *Diplostomulum xenopi* resides within the pericardial sac of *X laevis*. With chronic infection, fluid accumulates within the pericardial sac applying pressure on the lungs resulting in pulmonary distress. The distension of the pericardial sac also compresses the caval veins, reducing flow into the right atrium, decreasing ventricular output, and dropping systemic pressure eventually resulting in death. Hematoma formation occurs in some animals, affecting either the ventricular wall or epicardium. Cardiac tamponade has not been documented but pericardial adhesions to the body wall do occur.[34] *Clinostomum* spp are digenean trematodes that infect the lymph sacs and pericardial sacs of *X laevis* as well as hylid and ranid frogs.[35] This species uses both fish and amphibians as intermediate hosts.[36]

Other parasites affecting the amphibian cardiovascular system include trypanosomes, *Rhabdias* spp, and dipterans. Anuran trypanosome infection commonly affects the circulatory system leading to distension of lymph sacs with fluid and flagellates. *Trypanosoma inopinatum* is the best studied anuran trypanosome.[37] *Rhabdias* spp larvae migrate through heart muscle and frequently disperse hematogenously throughout the animal but particularly to the lungs.[38] Larvae can be detected in feces of infected amphibians. The dipterans *Batrachomyia* spp inhabit the dorsal lymph sacs of anurans. These fly larvae respire through spiracles accessing air through holes in the frog's skin. Frogs may survive infection or may succumb following larval emergence.[39]

CARDIOVASCULAR DISEASES: GENETIC AND IDIOPATHIC ETIOLOGIES

A variety of genetic and idiopathic etiologies of cardiovascular disease are known in laboratory-reared amphibians. Thrombosed, nonfunctional lymph hearts occur occasionally in laboratory-reared X laevis resulting in hydrops. The lymph spaces of these animals become markedly distended with fluid to such a degree that the frogs may double in size.[19] Affected animals may live for years but the edema never resolves and the animals fail to thrive.[40] Caudal edema trait or "caudal ascites" is a semi-lethal autosomal recessive disease of Spanish ribbed newt larvae (Pleurodeles waltl) resulting in tail edema.[41] An interesting phenomenon exploited by cardiovascular researchers is the "cardiac nonfunction" mutation (cardiac lethal gene c) of the Mexican axolotl (Ambystoma mexicanum). In homozygous recessive animals, there is incomplete cardiac differentiation resulting in a nonbeating heart and hydrops.[42] The exact nature of the defect is not characterized, although evidence suggests either a defect or absence of a component necessary for assembly of functional sarcomeric myofibrils such as tropomyosin.[43] Cardiac organogenesis is not affected and the mutant hearts are phenotypically indistinguishable from wild-type hearts until the heartbeat stage.[44] The mutant embryos live approximately 3 weeks after which the heart should have normally begun to beat, likely by simple diffusion of oxygen into tissues. Skeletal muscle is not affected by this mutation and swimming is normal. Transplantation of pre-heartbeat stage endoderm or extracted RNA from normal axolotls corrects the heart defect in the mutant axolotls.[45] Aortic and arterial atherosclerosis has been associated with the corneal lipidosis and xanthomatosis syndrome in captive tree frogs.[46] This syndrome is associated with an inappropriate high cholesterol diet and may occur at a higher incidence in females than male frogs.[47]

AMPHIBIANS AS CARDIOVASCULAR ANIMAL MODELS

Early work on the understanding of cardiovascular function was established from frog studies. These include the Nobel prize–winning work of August Krogh[48] on capillary regulation during rest and work. The Frank-Starling mechanism, the ability of the heart to alter contraction force and consequently stroke volume in response to alterations in venous return, the "Treppe" or staircase phenomenon, vagal nerve cardiac effects, cardiac dependence on oxidative metabolism, and other discoveries were all determined from experiments using isolated frog hearts.[49]

Amphibians have historically been a model for studying heart development because of the large size of their embryos, ease of breeding and maintaining animals, large numbers of larvae produced, transparency allowing visualization with surgical intervention, slow development amenable to manipulation, external development, and regenerative capacity.[42] Recent research has focused on urodele capacity for cardiac regeneration and the genes involved with the eventual goal of translating this information into therapies aimed at salvaging and repairing failing human hearts. Adult newts can survive the loss of 30% to 50% of the ventricle by dedifferentiation of adjacent undamaged cardiomyocytes and loss of intercalated discs. This is followed by DNA synthesis and mitosis of the cardiomyocytes and surrounding connective tissue. The defect is filled by fibrous scar tissue intermixed with a limited number of differentiated cardiomyocytes but does result in a functional heart.[50] Although this event represents a repair mechanism, it is not a complete or perfect regeneration of the heart damage. These data suggest that cardiomyocytes in the urodele are not terminally differentiated and can be prompted into proliferation.

VENIPUNCTURE

Commonly used venipuncture sites in anurans include the heart, ventral abdominal vein, femoral vein, and lingual vein. In salamanders, the ventral tail vein is the preferred site. In caecilians, cardiac puncture is the method of choice. In healthy amphibians, a blood volume of 1% of body weight is considered safe whereas in moribund animals, it is recommended not to exceed 0.5%. Lithium heparin is the optimal anticoagulant for amphibian blood samples.[17]

ACKNOWLEDGMENTS

A special thanks to Frank Taheny for the beautiful medical illustrations and Leigh Clayton and Kat Hadfield of the National Aquarium in Baltimore for providing the clinical photos and cytology.

REFERENCES

1. Sharma HL. The circulatory mechanism and anatomy of the heart of the frog, *Rana pipiens*. J Morphol 1961;109:323–49.
2. Staley NA, Benson ES. The ultrastructure of frog ventricular cardiac muscle and its relationship to mechanisms of excitation—contraction coupling. J Cell Biol 1968;38(1):99–114.
3. Zug GR, Vitt LJ, Caldwell JP. Herpetology: an introductory biology of amphibians and reptiles. 2nd edition. San Diego (CA): Academic Press; 2001.
4. Mohun TJ, Leong LM, Weninger WJ, et al. The morphology of heart development in *Xenopus laevis*. Dev Biol 2000;218:74–88.
5. Kolker SJ, Tajchman U, Weeks DL. Confocal imaging of early heart development in *Xenopus laevis*. Dev Biol 2000;218:64–73.
6. De Graaf AR. Investigations into the distribution of blood in the heart and the aortic arches of *Xenopus laevis* (Daud.). J Exp Biol 1957;34(2):143–72.
7. Duellman WE, Trueb L. Integumentary, sensory, and visceral systems. Biology of amphibians. Baltimore (MD): Johns Hopkins University Press; 1994. p. 670, xxi.
8. Putnam JL. Anatomy of the heart of the amphibia. I. *Siren lacertina*. Copeia 1977; 3:476–88.
9. Putnam JL, Kelly DL. A new interpretation of interatrial septation in the lungless salamander, *Plethodon glutinosus*. Copeia 1978;2:251–4.
10. Putnam JL, BP J. Anatomy of the heart of the amphibian. II. *Cryptobranchus alleganiensis*. Herpetologica 1985;41(3):287–98.
11. Putnam JL, Dunn JF. Septation in the ventricle of the heart of *Necturus maculosus*. Herpetologica 1978;34(3):292–7.
12. Putnam JL. Septation in ventricle of the heart of *Siren intermedia*. Copeia 1975;4: 773–4.
13. Nel NE. The anatomy of the heart of the plethodontid salamander *Ensatina eschscholtzii eschscholtzii* Gray. Annales Universitatis Stellenbosch 1970; A45(2):1–18.
14. Poupa O, Ostadal B. Experimental cardiomegalies and "cardiomegalies" in free-living animals. Ann N Y Acad Sci 1969;156:445–68.
15. Hillman SS. Cardiovascular correlates of maximal oxygen consumption rates in anuran amphibians. J Comp Physiol 1976;109:199–207.

16. Boutilier RG, Glass ML, Heisler N. The relative distribution of pulmocutaneous blood flow in *Rana catesbiana*: effects of pulmonary or cutaneous respiration. J Exp Biol 1986;126:33–9.

17. Wright KM. Anatomy for the clinician. In: Wright KM, Whitaker BR, editors. Amphibian medicine and captive husbandry. Original edition. Malabar (FL): Krieger Pub Co; 2001. p. 499, xxv.

18. Conklin RE. The formation and circulation of lymph in the frog: I. The rate of lymph production. Am J Physiol 1930;95:79–90.

19. Carter DB. Structure and function of the subcutaneous lymph sacs in the anura (Amphibia). J Herpetol 1979;13(3):321–7.

20. Drewes RC, Hedrick MS, Hillman SS, et al. Unique role of skeletal muscle contraction in vertical lymph movement in anurans. J Exp Biol 2007;210:3931–9.

21. Jolly JJ. Recherches sur le systeme lymphatique des batrachiens. Arch Anat Microsc Morphol Exp 1946;36:3–44.

22. Boutilier RG, Stiffler DF, Toews DP. Exchange of respiratory gases, ions, and water in amphibious and aquatic amphibians. In: Feder ME, Burggren WW, editors. Environmental physiology of the amphibians. Chicago (IL): University of Chicago Press; 1992. p. 81–124.

23. Lewis FM, Marsh BJ, Von Reyn CF. Fish tank exposure and cutaneous infections due to *Mycobacterium marinum*: tuberculin skin testing, treatment, and prevention. Clin Infect Dis 2003;37:390–7.

24. Bercovier H, Vincent V. Mycobacterial infections in domestic and wild animals due to *Mycobacterium marinum, M fortuitum, M chelonae, M porcinum, M farcinogenes, M smegmatis, M scrofulaceum, M xenopi, M kansasii, M simiae,* and *M genavense*. In: Collins MT, Manning B, editors. Mycobacterial infections in domestic and wild animals. Paris: Office International de Epizooties; 2001. p. 265–90.

25. Suykerbuyk P, Vleminckx K, Pasmans F, et al. *Mycobacterium lilandii* infection in European colony of *Silurana tropicalis*. Emerg Infect Dis 2007;13(5):743–6.

26. Bodetti TJ, Jacobson E, Wan C, et al. Molecular evidence to support the expansion of the hostrange of *Chlamydophila pneumoniae* to include reptiles, as well as humans, horses, koalas, and amphibians. Syst Appl Microbio 2002;25(1):146–52.

27. Blumer C, Zimmerman DR, Weilenmann R, et al. Chlamydiae in free-ranging and captive frogs in Switzerland. Vet Pathol 2007;44:144–50.

28. Howerth EW. Pathology of naturally occurring chlamydiosis in African clawed frogs (*Xenopus laevis*). Vet Pathol 1984;21(1):28–32.

29. Mok WY, Morato de Carvalho C. Association of anurans with pathogenic fungi. Mycopathologia 1985;92:37–43.

30. Speare R, Berger L, O'Shea P, et al. Pathology of mucormycosis of cane toads in Australia. J Wildl Dis 1997;33(1):105–11.

31. Hyatt AD, Parkes H, Zupanovic Z. Identification, characterisation and assessment of Venezuelan viruses for potential use as biological control agents against the cane toad (*Bufo marinus*) in Australia: Australian Federal Government and Environment Australia; 1998.

32. Docherty DE, Meteyer CU, Wang J, et al. Diagnostic and molecular evaluation of three iridovirus-associated salamander mortality events. J Wildl Dis 2003;39(3):556–66.

33. Bollinger TK, Mao J, Schock D, et al. Pathology, isolation, and preliminary molecular characterization of a novel iridovirus from tiger salamanders in Saskatchewan. J Wildl Dis 1999;35(3):413–29.

34. Nigrelli RF, Maraventano LW. Pericarditis in *Xenopus laevis* caused by *Diplostomulum xenopi* sp. nov., a larval strigeid. J Parasitol 1944;30(3):184–90.

35. Kuperman BI, Matey VE, Fisher RN, et al. Parasites of the African clawed frog, *Xenopus laevis*, in Southern California, USA. Comp Parasitol 2004;71(2):229–32.
36. Levine ND. Nematode parasites of domestic animals and of man. 2nd edition. Minneapolis (MN): Burgess Publishing; 1980.
37. Brumpt E. Un cas de rupture de la rate avec hemoperitoune au cors d'une infection experimentale a *Trypansoma inopinatum* chez la grenoulli verte (*Rana esculente*). Annales de Parasitologie 1924;4:325.
38. Williams RW. Observations on the life history of *Rhabdias sphaerocephala* Goodey, 1924 from *Bufo marinus* L., in the Bermuda Islands. J Helminthol 1960;34(1/2):93–8.
39. Elkan E. Miasis in Australian frogs. Ann Trop Med Parasitol 1965;59:51–4.
40. Balls M. The incidence of pathologic abnormalities, including spontaneous lymphosarcomas, in a laboratory stock of *Xenopus* (the South African clawed toad). Cancer Res 1965;25:3–6.
41. Beetschen JC, Jaylet A. On a semi-lethal recessive factor determining the appearance of caudal ascites (ac) in the triton *Pleurodeles waltii*. C R Hebd Seances Acad Sci Ser D Sci Nat 1965;261(25):5675–8.
42. Neff A, Dent AE, Armstrong JB. Heart development and regeneration in urodeles. Int J Dev Biol 1996;40:719–25.
43. Lemanski LF, Fuldner RA, Paulson DJ. Immunofluorescence studies for myosin, alpha-actinin, and tropomyosin in developing hearts of normal and cardiac lethal mutant Mexican axolotls, *Ambystoma mexicanum*. J Embryol Exp Morphol 1980; 55:1–15.
44. Lemanski LF. Morphology of developing heart in cardiac lethal mutant Mexican axolotls, *Ambystoma mexicanum*. Dev Biol 1973;33:312–33.
45. Lemanski LF, Paulson DJ, Hill GS. Normal anterior endoderm corrects the heart defect in cardiac mutant salamanders (*Ambystoma mexicanum*). Science 1979;204:860–2.
46. Carpenter JL, Bachrach A, Albert DM, et al. Xanthomatous keratitis, disseminated xanthomatosis, and atherosclerosis in Cuban tree frogs. Vet Pathol 1986;23(3): 337–9.
47. Shilton CM, Smith DA, Crawshaw GJ, et al. Corneal lipid deposition in Cuban tree frogs (*Osteopilus septentrionalis*) and its relationship to serum lipids: an experimental study. J Zoo Wildl Med 2001;32(3):305–19.
48. Krogh A. Studies on the capillariometer mechanism: I. The reaction to stimuli and the innervation of the blood vessels in the tongue of the frog. J Physiol 1920;53(6): 399–419.
49. Zimmer HG. Modifications of the isolated frog heart preparation in Carl Ludwig's Leipzig Physiological Institute: relevance for cardiovascular research. Can J Cardiol 2000;16(1):61–9.
50. Oberpriller JO, Oberpriller JC. Response of the adult newt ventricle to injury. J Exp Zool 1974;187:248–60.

Normal Reptile Heart Morphology and Function

Jeanette Wyneken, PhD

KEYWORDS

- Myocardium • Ventricle • Atrium • Cardiac • Muscular ridge
- Cavum arteriosum • Cavum venosum • Vacum pulmonale

Reptile hearts are simple in their external gross morphology but are complex internally. The reptilian heart structure that is often described to introductory biology students is deceptively simple because of the conceptual framework in which it is presented. Even today, organ systems are described erroneously as though representing steps in a linear progression from simple to increasingly complex and sophisticated vertebrates. In this stepwise linear framework, the relatively simple tubular fish heart is at the base, the four-chambered mammalian heart is at the top, and the hearts of amphibians (three chambers) and reptiles (three chambers, with a complex ventricle) form other steps. Such an orderly sequential perspective dates back to Aristotle, who tried to understand the complexity of organisms by arranging them hierarchically as a "Ladder of Life" (*scala naturae*) based on structure. Such views of morphological diversity ignore the branching and tree-like histories of organisms. The diversity of vertebrate heart forms, including those found in reptiles, are best viewed in the context of diverse and nonlinear histories with many different branches.

Reptilian heart anatomy varies around a few major structural patterns. Although each design appears grossly to have two atria and a single ventricle, there is much more to this system, which reflects the physiological demands and lifestyles of the animals. In many cases, structural-functional features of the reptilian heart clearly are adaptive to the ecology and behavior of the species. It is the structure of the systems that provides the functional plasticity. The circulatory and respiratory systems are structurally and functionally related in all vertebrates and are often discussed together as the cardiopulmonary system. This review focuses on the heart and great vessels (cardiovascular anatomy), however, and omits the peripheral circulation and the pulmonary components.

Department of Biological Sciences, 266 Building 01, Sanson Science, Florida Atlantic University, 777 Glades Road, Boca Raton, FL 33431–0991 USA
E-mail address: jwyneken@fau.edu

Vet Clin Exot Anim 12 (2009) 51–63
doi:10.1016/j.cvex.2008.08.001
1094-9194/08/$ – see front matter © 2009 Elsevier Inc. All rights reserved.

COMPARATIVE HEART SHAPE, SIZE, AND LOCATION

The hearts of snakes are elongate, whereas those of chelonians, crocodilians, lizards, and tuataras tend to be more ovoid or triangular in shape (**Figs. 1** and **2**). Heart mass is 0.20% to 0.32% of body mass in reptiles, with proportionately larger hearts found in more athletic species and in climbing snakes.[1]

The location of the heart varies within reptilian lineages and even within taxa, although the heart tends to be positioned roughly along the axial midline. In chelonians, part of the heart is often deep to margins of the humeral and pectoral scutes; however, in some species, it is positioned more posteriorly along the midline between humeral-pectoral and pectoral-abdominal scute lines.[2] In soft-shelled turtles (Trionychidae), the heart is displaced to the right.[1] The shoulder girdles provide good landmarks in radiographs; the heart is typically just caudal to the level of the acromion processes and cranial to the distal procoracoid process–procoracoid cartilage junction.

In lizards, the heart position may approach the gular regions (geckos of the genus *Hemidactylus*[1] and bearded dragons [*Pogona vitticeps*]) or may occur more caudally within the rib cage (chameleons, iguanas, and varanids). In adult or large immature iguanid and varanid lizards, the caudal portion of the ventricle is aligned with the elbow when the arms are retracted against the body. In younger lizards, the heart may fill much of the thoracic cavity, extending from the elbow level cranially to just posterior to the axilla.

In most snakes, the heart is found at a position that is located from 22% to 33% of the snout-vent length (15%–25% of total length) caudal to the rostrum. The heart is often shifted caudally, in totally aquatic snakes, to a position that ranges from 25% to 45% of total length caudal to the rostrum.[1–3] Differences in heart position in boids, elapids, crotalids, and colubrids are described by McCracken.[4]

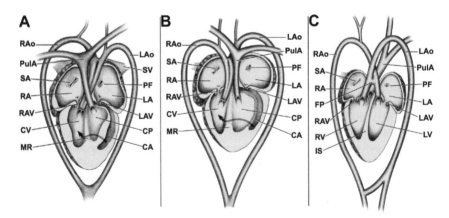

Fig. 1. Diagrams of reptilian heart structure, including chambers, compartments, and great vessels, comparing the turtles and general squamate pattern (*A*), varanid pattern (*B*), and that of crocodilians (*C*). The pulmonary artery (= pulmonary trunk) arises as a single structure then bifurcates. *Abbreviations*: CA, cavum arteriosum; CP, cavum pulmonale; CV, cavum venosum; FP, foramen of Panizza; IS, interventricular septum; LA, left atrium; LAo, left aorta; LAV, left atrioventricular valve; LV, left ventricle; MR, muscular ridge; PF, pulmonary vein foramen; PulA, pulmonary artery; RA, right atrium; RAo, right aorta; RAV, right atrioventricular valve; RV, right ventricle; SA, sinoatrial valve; SV, sinus venosus (*Courtesy of* Jeanette Wyneken, PhD, Boca Raton, FL).

COMPARATIVE HEART ANATOMY

Reptilian cardiovascular anatomy varies with taxon. Reptilian hearts are described here by major structural patterns within taxonomic contexts. Chambers or compartments of noncrocodilian ventricles are usually morphologically connected so that systemic and pulmonary circuits share space. When necessary, the author describes structures functionally by the relative condition of blood's oxygenation (high or low oxygen content of blood).

PERICARDIAL ANATOMY

The heart is located within the pericardium. The pericardial sac typically contains clear pericardial fluid that, at least in turtles, is rich in calcium and magnesium ions. The alkaline pericardial fluid that bathes the heart may play a minor role in protection from acidosis during apnea.[5] In some reptiles, the caudal aspect of the pericardium and apex of the ventricle are attached to the visceral peritoneum by a cord-like ligament, the gubernaculum cordis. This structure is present in most chelonians, most lizards, tuataras, and crocodilians but is absent in snakes and varanid lizards.[1,6,7] When present, the structure anchors the ventricle so that longitudinal tension may be developed during contraction. Anchoring one possible mechanism by which the muscular walls and ridges may functionally divide the ventricle during contraction rather than retracting the ventricle craniad.[8]

GROSS CARDIAC ANATOMY

The reptilian heart is more complex than its exterior betrays. It is composed of five or six chambers and compartments: the sinus venosus, the left and right atria, and two or three subchambers or compartments of the ventricle. There are three basic patterns of reptilian heart structure (see **Fig. 1**); most squamates (lizards and snakes), chelonians, and rhynchocephalians (tuataras) share one form; varanid lizards and pythons show variants that may be viewed as a second pattern; and another is found in crocodilians.[1,8–10]

SINUS VENOSUS

The first chamber to receive systemic blood in all reptiles is the sinus venosus; this thin sac-like structure is often ignored when chambers are described and counted.[2] It can be large, although it is usually smaller than the combined volume of the atria and ventricle, and is located dorsal to the atria and ventricle.[1] The walls are formed of cardiac muscle and connective tissues. The sinus venosus is undivided in chelonians and tuataras; an incomplete septum partially divides it in squamates and crocodilians.[1]

Venous blood from the body drains into the sinus venosus from four major veins: the left precava (left superior vena cava), the right precava (right superior vena cava), the left hepatic vein, and the postcava (posterior vena cava). The sinus venosus is connected to the muscular right atrium by way of a sinoatrial aperture.

ATRIOVENTRICULAR ANATOMY IN SQUAMATES, CHELONIANS, AND RHYNCHOCEPHALIANS

The hearts of turtles, most lizards, and snakes have two atria and one ventricle (see **Figs. 1** and **2**); the ventricle is partitioned into interconnected subchambers or compartments.[1,10,11] The left atrium is separate from the right atrium and tends to be smaller and less muscular. The left atrium receives blood from the pulmonary vein by way of an opening, which may be exposed or may be guarded against backflow by

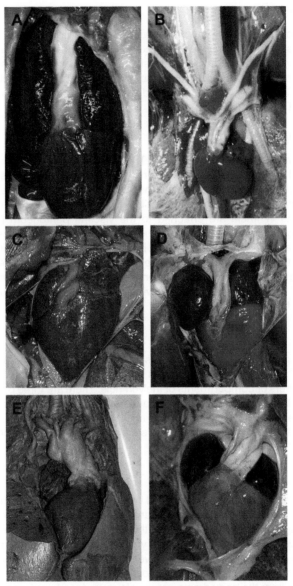

Fig. 2. Ventral views of several adult or subadult reptilian hearts, including a Burmese python (*Python molurus*) (*A*), slider turtle (*Trachemys scripta*) (*B*), green iguana (*Iguana iguana*) (*C*), bearded dragon (*Pogona vitticeps*) (*D*), and American alligator (*Alligator mississippiensis*) (*E*). Heart of a neonate sea turtle (*Dermochelys coriacea*) (*F*) shows the relatively short rounded ventricle anchored at its apex to the pericardial sac. (*Courtesy of* J. Wyneken, PhD, Boca Raton, FL.)

a loose flap-like fold of the atrial wall (a pulmoatrial valve). The atria communicate with the ventricle by way of atrioventricular funnels.[1,8] The ventricle of most squamates, chelonians, and the tuataras is comprised of three interconnected compartments or "subchambers:" the cavum pulmonale, cavum venosum, and cavum arteriosum (see **Fig. 1**). The cavum arteriosum and cavum venosum are located mostly dorsal to the cavum pulmonale.

Within the ventricle of noncrocodilian reptiles, there is a muscular septum that starts immediately caudal to the interatrial septum and extends toward the apex, but it is unattached to the ventral wall of the ventricle through much of its length and so does not fully separate the ventricle. It partially separates the cavum arteriosum and the cavum venosum and functionally seems to separate pulmonary and systemic blood flow. Additionally, noncrocodilian reptiles have a muscular ridge arising from the base of the aortae and extending along the dorsal wall toward the ventricular apex. This muscular ridge is poorly developed in most chelonians but is well developed in many squamates, particularly varanids and pythons.[1,6]

The subchambers may be easiest to understand in the context of blood flow within the ventricle (and without intracardiac shunting, as discussed elsewhere in this article). Both atria supply blood to the ventricle simultaneously (**Fig. 3**). The right atrium supplies blood to the cavum venosum, whereas blood flows into the cavum arteriosum from the left atrium.[1,9,10] The cavum pulmonale receives blood from the cavum venosum. During ventricular systole, blood can exit to the circulation from the cavum pulmonale and the cavum venosum. Blood leaving the cavum pulmonale primarily flows to the pulmonary artery and then to the lungs. Blood flows from the cavum venosum to the aortic trunk; from there, it goes to the head and body. Blood from the cavum pulmonale also may enter the left aorta (see **Fig. 3**). Blood cannot leave the cavum arteriosum directly; its blood passes through an interventricular canal to the cavum

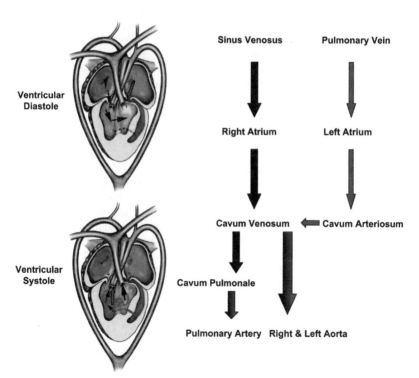

Fig. 3. Diagram of blood flow through a noncrocodlian reptile heart. No intracardiac shunting is shown. Blood normally flows among the ventricular compartments as shown by arrows. Red indicates high oxygen blood; blue indicates low oxygen blood.

venosum. The cavum venosum and cavum pulmonale are continuous with one another during diastole; thus, any separation of high and low oxygen blood must be maintained by blood flow streams rather than by physical separation. During ventricular contraction, the cava venosum and cava pulmonale become separated by a muscular ridge that occludes the intervening space.

HEARTS OF VARANID LIZARDS AND PYTHONS

In varanid lizards (monitors) and pythons, the ventricle still consists of three subchambers but differs morphologically in that each can separate blood flow functionally into pulmonary and systemic circuits. In varanids, the cavum arteriosum is large compared with that of other reptiles and the cavum venosum is reduced (see **Fig. 1**).[1] The ventricle creates some separation between high and low oxygen blood and systemic and pulmonary outflow, because asymmetry in wall thickness creates a pressure differential between the right and left sides and a muscular ridge functionally divides the heart into pulmonary and systemic circuits during systole.[1,12–16] As in other noncrocodilian reptiles, blood from the cavum pulmonale leaves the varanid heart by way of the pulmonary artery and blood flows into to the systemic aortae from the cavum venosum.[1]

In pythons, the ventricle's three subchambers do not show the size asymmetry found in varanids. The cavum arteriosum is most dorsal and is separated from the cavum venosum and cavum pulmonale by an incomplete muscular partition, the interventricular septum (also termed *horizontal septum*). An interventricular canal allows blood from the cavum arteriosum to enter into the cavum venosum. Blood moving between the cavum venosum and cavum pulmonale passes a well-developed muscular ridge. As contraction occurs, the atrioventricular valves direct blood flow from the right and left atria into the cavum venosum and cavum arteriosum, respectively. The muscular ridge functionally divides the heart into pulmonary and systemic circuits during systole; thus, blood flows as separate streams to the cavum pulmonale and cavum venosum, respectively.[1,7,15,17] In this way, high oxygen blood enters the left and right aortae from the cavum venosum, whereas lower oxygen blood from the cavum pulmonale flows into the pulmonary trunk.

HEARTS OF CROCODILIANS

The heart in crocodilians has two atria and a ventricle that is physically divided into pulmonary and systemic circuits.[1,8] This cardiac structure is grossly reminiscent of that of birds and mammals, except for the presence of left and right aortic arches.[13] The atria are similar in size; the interventricular septum is fully developed in crocodilians, such that the ventricle is structurally and functionally divided into two chambers (right and left ventricles) (see **Fig. 1**).[1,9] Blood from the right ventricle flows into the pulmonary trunk and the left aorta. Blood from the left ventricle flows into the right aorta. The two aortae are interconnected near the heart by the foramen of Panizza and slightly distal to the heart by the dorsal connecting artery,[1] which is rostral to the convergence of the two systemic aortae as the single dorsal aorta.

VALVES

The reptilian heart has valves and a ventricular muscular ridge that, together, separate subchambers and control the direction of blood flow. The sinoatrial valve is formed by flaps of endocardium that overlie one another and separate the sinus venosus from the right atrium. In all reptiles, the left atrium receives blood through a valve-free opening at the base of the pulmonary vein. In squamates, chelonians, and tuataras, the atrioventricular valves are variously described as bell-shaped,[9] single-cusped,[13] or having multiple cusps varying in size (small marginal cusps).[1] They direct blood into the cavum venosum and the venosum pulmonale during atrial systole and prevent regurgitation of blood into the atria during ventricular systole. The bases of the aortae have bicuspid valves, and in most reptiles, the base of the pulmonary trunk has semilunar valves.[1] The bicuspid atrioventricular valves of crocodilians lead from the two atria to the two ventricles separated by the muscular septum.[1,9] In crocodilians, blood leaving the right ventricle during ventricular systole passes by paired lobe-like valves, which fit together like cogs to regulate blood flow into the pulmonary artery. The bicuspid valves at the bases of the aortae are asymmetric in size, with the larger cusps occurring on the aortic septal sides.[9]

MYOCARDIUM

The walls of the sinus venosus are formed by connective tissues with some myocytes; the atrial walls all contain connective tissues (elastic and fibrous) but have a much greater proportion formed by myocytes. The ventricle is primarily muscular with the least connective tissue; its walls are formed by three muscle layers.[1] A thin muscular layer of longitudinally arranged myocytes overlies the spirally arranged myocytes of the compact myocardium. Internal to the compact layer is spongy myocardium that also forms the trabeculae. The density of the spongy trabeculae varies within taxa and across the Reptilia. Species with narrow hearts tend to have fewer trabecular ridges, whereas those that have round or short ventricles have many (eg, marine turtles).[1] In young animals and tuataras, the compact layer is poorly developed.[1]

GREAT VESSELS

The great vessels are the three major arteries that emerge from the cranial and ventral parts of the ventricle: the left aorta, the right aorta, and a pulmonary trunk (see **Fig. 1**). These three vessels and their tributaries have thick, muscular, and elastic walls and are typically "high-pressure" vessels. The bases of the aortae, including the interaortic septum, are supported by cartilage; in older animals, this cartilage may normally be calcified.[1,11,15] The gross configuration of the great vessels varies with taxa. The aortae of chelonians tend to have particularly large bases when compared with those of other reptiles and arise dorsally and slightly to the right of the pulmonary trunk.

The left aorta arches dorsally and to the left as it travels caudally in the body, giving off several smaller arteries to the abdominal viscera before joining the right aorta to form the dorsal aorta. The right aorta arches dorsally and slightly to the right and then travels caudally and gives off major branches that supply blood to the head, stomach, pancreas, spleen, and duodenum before joining the left aorta. The pulmonary trunk gives rise to the right and left pulmonary arteries to the right and left lungs.

In squamates, chelonians, and tuatara, the aortic trunk, formed of the bases of the left and right aortae, seems to arise from the midline or right side of the ventricle. The pulmonary trunk arises from the cranial part of the ventricle. In monitor lizards, the left aorta arises slightly more ventrally than the pulmonary trunk.[12] In iguanas (*Iguana iguana*), the left aorta and pulmonary trunk arise cranioventrally but show variable levels of torsion, such that their paths quickly become circuitous.[16] In the tuatara, the paired aortae exit the ventricle by way of an elevated muscular conus arteriosus located to the right of the midline.[8]

A semilunar valve controls flow between the ventricle and the base of the aortae. Blood leaving the ventricle tends to separate into systemic and pulmonary flow or may be directed to just systemic flow by passing along a series of muscular ridges in the ventricle. In some species, the flow of blood to a pulmonary or systemic path may be regulated by asymmetry in the ventricular contraction.[1,18]

CARDIOPULMONARY CIRCULATION

The reptile heart is not uniform in the supply and position of its coronary arteries and veins. Well-developed coronary vessel systems supply the compact myocardium on the left and right sides of the heart.[19] The heart's spongy muscle receives oxygenated blood as it passes through the chambers and compartments.[18] In pythons, the coronary arteries are particularly concentrated in the atria and the cavum arteriosum.[19]

The extent of separation of the pulmonary and systemic circuits of flow is directed, in part, by a muscular ridge within the ventricle and by blood flow streams.[20] The details of intraventricular structure differ across taxa as described previously, and flow paths are often inferred from physiologic data. The importance of the form of the ventricle's muscular ridge in directing flow and separating high and low oxygen blood has an extensive literature.[10-15,17,18] The muscular ridge is relatively small in freshwater chelonian species, such as *Trachemys*, but more robust in animals that are large active divers, such as sea turtles, and in giant tortoises.[1,11] Although several reptilian species have been studied,[1,21] there are relatively few experimental studies that define the heart's structural and functional relationships[13,14,21-30] and fewer yet that are comparative.[15,25,27] Most work has focused on crocodilians.[9,31] Within squamates, relatively few species have been studied, with varanids and pythons[12-14,28,29] receiving the most attention. The clinician should note that extrapolation of cardiac structure and performance from these large-bodied, specialized animals to taxonomically more distant species may not be appropriate.

Circulation through the heart differs depending on whether blood is shunted toward the lungs and the body or primarily toward the body. Unlike mammalian cardiovascular systems, the pulmonary and systemic blood flows are not morphologically separated into fully parallel circuits. The extent of separation between the pulmonary and systemic blood flows differs within reptiles as the result of the several different structural patterns, including separate ventricles in crocodilians,[9,15,26,27] and the degree of intraventricular septum and muscular ridge development.[21,29,30] Even within turtles, which usually have limited development of the ventricle's muscular ridge, some separation of high and low oxygen blood flow may occur.[1,6,23] Flow separation may be linked to structure more clearly in the largest chelonian species. For example, the leatherback sea turtle (*Dermochelys coriacea*) has an exceptionally well-developed muscular ridge and well-developed muscular sphincters controlling flow to the pulmonary arteries. These blood flow–directing structures are moderately well developed in other marine turtles[6,32] and Galapagos tortoises (*Geochelone elephantopus*).[1,33]

CARDIAC SHUNTS

Cardiac shunts are patterns of intraventricular blood flow and require an incomplete septum; these are found in noncrocodilian reptiles. Shunts are often described as "right to left" (R-L), referring to the shift in blood from the pulmonary circulation to the body (the system) alone, and "left to right" (L-R), referring to the shift of blood back to the lungs and the body when physiologic conditions permit.[21] During normal resting reptilian ventilation, the flow of blood tends to create a L-R shunt based on pressure differentials. During ventricular systole, blood flows to the systemic and pulmonary circuits.[22] During diving, apnea, or other instances in which the pulmonary resistance can elevate, a R-L shunt may occur (in crocodilian, a similar event is a pulmonary-to-systemic shunt described elsewhere in this article).[21–25,27–31] This means that flow to the pulmonary arteries is reduced and most blood exiting the ventricle shifts to the systemic vessels. Low systemic blood oxygen levels resulting from large-scale R-L shunting may serve to regulate metabolism.[32] When any of several physiologic events or environmental factors (temperature, exercise, or digestion) increase metabolism, the R-L cardiac shunt reduces and oxygen delivery to the lungs increases. Many reptiles are able to function at much lower Po_2 levels and higher Pco_2 levels than mammals. Reptilian species that are able to sustain the highest metabolic rates tend to possess the highest degree of anatomic ventricular separation and, therefore, less cardiac shunting. In addition to regulating blood gas levels,[33] intracardiac shunts also play an important role in oxygenating the myocardium in the freshwater turtle (Trachemys scripta).[23]

Vagal tone is also correlated with development and regulation of L-R shunts.[8,33] The aortae and pulmonary trunk receive vagal innervation. Studies of turtles generally show that whether blood is shunted to or away from the lungs is a function of blood arterial gas levels; low systemic Po_2 tends to result in L-R shunt development; however, multiple factors may influence control.[34,35] For example, environmental factors, such as temperature, or other metabolic demands may reduce or reverse the shunt.[26,27,33] Anesthesia agents, such as propranolol, that block cholinergically mediated constriction of pulmonary arteries result in large L-R shunts.[36]

Several valve types are associated with the development of high pulmonary outflow resistance during apnea. Sphincters are found in the pulmonary arteries of marine turtles (Caretta caretta, Chelonia mydas, and Dermochelys coriacea); their constriction or relaxation seems to promote intracardiac shunting.[6,11,37]

Although crocodilians lack intraventricular shunting, the origins of the aortae in separate ventricles and the foramen of Panizza between the two aortae may serve a similar function.[27,28,32] The cog-shaped valve at the base of the pulmonary artery controls blood flow to the pulmonary circulation by phased closing during ventricular systole.[38] During normal ventilation, the pulmonary and systemic blood flows are separate in crocodilians. During apnea or diving, pulmonary flow is restricted by vasoconstriction of the pulmonary artery, resulting in mixing of oxygenated and deoxygenated blood in the left aorta by way of the foramen of Panizza, and possibly the connecting artery.

CONDUCTION

Reptile hearts lack the specialized Purkinje fiber–based conduction or "pacemaker" system found in mammals. Contraction is initiated by the cardiac muscle fibers in the sinus venosus,[1] and sequential coordination of chamber contraction is accomplished by the myofiber arrangements within and surrounding the openings of each chamber.[1] Ventricular systole tends to be long, and diastole is short. Reptilian electrocardiograms (ECGs) are grossly similar to those of mammals with P, QRS, and T complexes.[39] An SV wave from the sinus venosus (and postcava) may be measured just before the P wave. Probe position and temperature can affect reptilian ECGs.[40] In animals examined within their normal range of environmental temperature, the QT interval may be elongated and the interval between the T wave and the next P wave can be short.

HEART RATE

Reptilian heart rates are notoriously variable. Heart rates change with temperature (increasing, sometimes dramatically, during basking and lowering during cooling, which is termed *heart rate hysteresis*),[41,42] body size (slower in smaller reptiles),[1] activity (increasing heart rate with activity),[43,44] respiration (faster during ventilation, slower during apnea),[1] digestion, and pregnancy.[41,42] The heart rate in freshwater turtles (*T scripta*) nearly doubles during ventilation (from the resting rate during apnea).[45] "Diving bradycardia" is well known in many vertebrates, including reptiles, but is not restricted to submergence events.[41] Handling is known to increase heart rate in the green iguana (*Iguana iguana*).[46]

The vagus nerve innervates the reptile heart.[8,34] Well-developed vagal parasympathetic fibers provide cholinergic (inhibitory) control, and less well-developed sympathetic fibers modulate heart rate by androgenic (cardioaccelerator) fibers.[1,47–49]

PRESSURES

Most blood pressure measurements for reptiles are based on physiologic studies using invasive (surgically placed) pressure transducers. Great vessel pressures have been determined by direct intra-arterial means in several reptile species during rest or activity;[1,3,12,15,17,30,31,50] however, how these measurements might relate to clinical measures is unclear. One small study of three boid snakes (*Boa constrictor*) attempted to relate measures of blood pressure taken with surgically placed arterial pressure probes (direct blood pressure determination) to those obtained using pressure cuffs on the tail and connected to an oscillometric blood pressure monitor (indirect blood pressure determination). Indirect blood pressure measurements tended to underestimate diastolic pressure and mean arterial blood pressure but overestimated systolic arterial pressure.[40] Hence, at this time, additional simultaneous measures of blood pressure by clinical means in combination with direct intra-arterial pressure measurements are needed for most reptile taxa.

CLINICAL OVERVIEW

Several clinical overviews address various aspects of reptile cardiovascular morphology and function.[2,51–53] This article updates clinical context, provides discussion of the morphological varieties of reptilian cardiovascular systems, and highlights the functional implications to facilitate the assessment and treatment of reptile patients.

REFERENCES

1. Farrell AP, Graperil AK, Frances ETB. Comparative aspects of heart morphology. In: Gans C, Gaunt AS, editors. Biology of the Reptilia, Visceral organs, vol. 19. New York: Society for the Study of Amphibians and Reptiles; 1998. p. 375–424.
2. Kik MJL, Mitchell MA. Reptile cardiology: a review of anatomy and physiology, diagnostic approaches, and clinical disease. Semin Avian Exot Pet Med 2005; 14(1):52–60.
3. Seymour R. Scaling of cardiovascular physiology in snakes. Integr Comp Biol 1987;27:97–109.
4. McCracken HE. Organ location in snakes for diagnostic and surgical evaluation. In: Miller RE, editor. Zoo and wildlife medicine, current therapy 4. Philadelphia: W.B. Saunders; 1999. p. 243–8.
5. Jackson DC, Heisler N. The contribution of the alkaline pericardial fluid of freshwater turtles to acid buffering during prolonged anoxia. J Exp Biol 1984;109: 55–62.

6. Wyneken J. The structure of cardiopulmonary systems of turtles: implications for behavior. In: Wyneken J, Godfrey M, Bels V, editors. The biology of turtles. Boca Raton: CRC Press; 2008. p. 213–24.

7. Webb GJW, Heatwole H, de Bavay J. Comparative cardiac anatomy of the Reptilia. I. The chambers and septa of the varanid ventricle. J Morphol 1971; 134:335–50.

8. Webb GJW, Heatwole H, de Bavay J. Comparative cardiac anatomy of the Reptilia. II. A critique of the literature on the Squamata and Rhynchocephalia. J Morphol 1974;142:1–20.

9. Webb GJW. Comparative cardiac anatomy of the Reptilia. III. The heart of crocodilians and an hypothesis on the completion of the interventricular septum of crocodilians and birds. J Morphol 1979;161:221–40.

10. Kardong KV. Vertebrates: comparative anatomy, function, evolution. 4th edition. Boston: McGraw-Hill; 2006.

11. Wyneken J. Guide to the anatomy of sea turtles. NOAA Tech., Memo NMFS-SEFSC-470. Miami (FL): NMFS technical publication; 2001.

12. Heisler N, Neumann P, Maloiy GMO. The mechanism of intracardiac shunting in the lizard Varanus exanthematicus. J Exp Biol 1983;105:15–31.

13. Wang T, Altimiras J, Axelsson M. Intracardiac flow separation in an in situ perfused heart of Burmese python Python molurus. J Exp Biol 2002;205:2715–23.

14. Wang T, Altimiras J, Klein W, et al. Ventricular haemodynamics in Python molurus: separation of pulmonary and systemic pressures. J Exp Biol 2003;206:4241–5.

15. Burggren WW. Form and function in reptilian circulations. Am Zool 1987;27(1): 5–19.

16. Oldman JC, Smith M. Laboratory anatomy of the iguana. Dubuque (IA): William C. Brown Company; 1975.

17. White FN. Functional anatomy of the heart of reptiles. Am Zool 1968;8:211–9.

18. Zaar M, Overgaard J, Gesser H, et al. Contractile properties of the functionally divided python heart: two sides of the same matter. Comp Biochem Physiol A Mol Integr Physiol 2007;146:163–73.

19. MacKinnon MR, Heatwole H. Comparative cardiac anatomy of the Reptilia. IV. The coronary arterial circulation. J Morphol 1981;170:1–27.

20. Van Mierop LHS, Kutsche LM. Some aspects of comparative anatomy of the heart. In: Johansen K, Burggren W, editors. Alfred Benzon symposium 21: cardiovascular shunts: phylogenetic, ontogenetic and clinical aspects. Copenhagen: Munksgaard; 1985. p. 38–53.

21. Hicks JW. Cardiac shunting in reptiles: mechanisms, regulation and physiological function. In: Gans C, Gaunt AS, editors. Biology of the Reptilia. Ithaca, NY: Society for the Study of Amphibians and Reptiles; 1998. p. 425–83.

22. Farmer CG, Hicks JW. The intracardiac shunt as a source of myocardial oxygen in a turtle, Trachemys scripta. Integr Comp Biol 2002;42:208–15.

23. Hicks JW, Wang T. Functional role of cardiac shunts in reptiles. J Exp Zool 1996; 275:204–16.

24. Sapsford CW. Anatomical evidence for intracardiac blood shunting in marine turtles. Afr Zool 1978;13(1):57–62.

25. Burggren WW, Shelton G. Gas exchange and transport during intermittent breathing in chelonian reptiles. J Exp Biol 1979;82:75–92.

26. Burggren WW. The pulmonary circulation of the chelonian reptile: morphology, pharmacology and haemodynamics. J Comp Physiol [B] 1977;116:303–24.

27. Shelton G, Burggren WW. Cardiovascular dynamics of the Chelonia during apnoea and lung ventilation. J Exp Biol 1976;64:323–43.

28. Jones DR. The crocodilian central circulation: reptilian or avian? Verh Zool Bot Ges Wien 1996;89:209–18.

29. Jones DR, Shelton G. The physiology of the alligator heart: left aortic flow patterns and right-to-left shunts. J Exp Biol 1993;176:247–69.

30. Burggren WW, Johansen K. Ventricular haemodynamics in the monitor lizard *Varanus exanthematicus*: pulmonary and systemic pressure separation. J Exp Biol 1982;96:343–54.

31. Axelsson M, Franklin CE. From anatomy to angioscopy: 164 years of crocodilian cardiovascular research, recent advances, and speculations. Comp Biochem Physiol A Physiol 1997;118(1):51–62.

32. White FN. Circulation. In: Gans C, Dawson ER, editors. Biology of the Reptilia. New York: Academic Press; 1976. p. 275–334.

33. Wang T, Krosniunasi EH, Hicks JW. The role of cardiac shunts in the regulation of arterial blood gases. Am Zool 1997;37(1):12–22.

34. Wang T, Warburton S, Abe A, et al. Vagal control of heart rate and cardiac shunts in reptiles: relation to metabolic state. Exp Physiol 2001;86(6):777–84.

35. Porges SW, Riniolo TC, McBride T, et al. Heart rate and respiration in reptiles: contrasts between a sit-and-wait predator and an intensive forager. Brain Cogn 2003;52:88–96.

36. Overgaard J, Stecyk JAW, Farrell AP, et al. Adrenergic control of the cardiovascular system in the turtle *Trachemys scripta*. J Exp Biol 2002;205(13):3335–45.

37. Koch W. Lungengefässe und Kreislauf der Schildkröten. Biologia Gen (Vienna) 1934;10:359–82 [in German].

38. Syme DA, Gamperl K, Jones DRT. Delayed depolarization of the cog-wheel valve and pulmonary-to-systemic shunting in alligators. J Exp Biol 2002;205(13):1843–51.

39. Farrell AP. Circulation in vertebrates. Encyclopedia of life sciences. Chichester (UK): Nature Publishing Group; 2001. p. 1–15.

40. Chinnadurai SK, Devoe RS. Validation of oscillometric non-invasive blood pressure monitoring in boid snakes. Proceedings of the AAZV, AAWV, AZA/NAG Joint Conference. 2007. p. 61–2.

41. Seebacher F. Heat transfer in a microvascular network: the effect of heart rate on heating and cooling in reptiles (*Pogona barbata* and *Varanus varius*). J Theor Biol 2000;03(2):97–109.

42. Franklin CE, Seebacher F. The effect of heat transfer mode on heart rate responses and hysteresis during heating and cooling in the estuarine crocodile *Crocodylus porosus*. J Exp Biol 2003;206:1143–51.

43. Munns SL, Hartzler LK, Bennett AF, et al. Terrestrial locomotion does not constrain venous return in the American alligator, *Alligator mississippiensis*. J Exp Biol 2005;208:3331–9.

44. Munns SL, Hartzler LK, Bennett AF, et al. Elevated intra-abdominal pressure limits venous return during exercise in *Varanus exanthematicus*. J Exp Biol 2004; 207(23):4111–20.

45. Galli G, Taylor EW, Wang T. The cardiovascular responses of the freshwater turtle *Trachemys scripta* to warming and cooling. J Exp Biol 2004;207:1471–8.

46. Cabanac A, Cabanac M. Heart rate response to gentle handling of frog and lizard. Behav Processes 2000;52(2–3):89–95.

47. Berger PJ, Burnstock G. Autonomic nervous system. In: Gans C, Northcutt RG, Ulinski P, editors. Biology of the Reptilia, (Neurology B). vol. 10. Chicago: University of Chicago Press; 1979. p. 1–57.

48. Burnstock G. Evolution of the autonomic innervation of visceral and cardiovascular systems in vertebrates. Pharmacol Rev 1969;21:247–324.

49. Crossley DA II, Wang T, Altimiras J. Role of nitric oxide in the systemic and pulmonary circulation of anesthetized turtles (*Trachemys scripta*). J Exp Zool 2000; 86:683–9.

50. Jackson DC. Cardiovascular function in turtles during anoxia and acidosis: in vivo and in vitro studies. Am Zool 1987;27(1):49–58.

51. Williams DL. Cardiovascular system. In: Beynon PH, Lawton MPC, Cooper JE, editors. Manual of reptiles. Cheltenham (UK): British Small Animal Veterinary Association; 1992. p. 80–7.

52. Murray MJ. Cardiology. In: Mader DR, editor. Reptile medicine and surgery. 2nd edition. Philadelphia: WB Saunders/Elsevier; 2006. p. 181–95.

53. Wyneken J. The anatomy of reptiles. Krieger Publishing Company, Inc., in press.

Reptile Cardiology

Mark A. Mitchell, DVM, MS, PhD

KEYWORDS

• Blood • Cardiology • Heart • Reptile • Vascular

To date, clinical reptile cardiology is a field that has received limited attention. Veterinarians should not find this surprising, however, because the cardiology specialty in the American College of Veterinary Internal Medicine is small (with fewer than 200 diplomates), and most of the research being pursued by these individuals is related to domestic species. Although clinical research related to the field is limited, a large body of literature related to the physiologic and evolutionary importance of reptile cardiology is available.[1] Because of the small body of clinical evidence related to the field, it is important that veterinarians apply that knowledge that is available in managing clinical cases.

The clinical relevance of cardiology for reptiles remains an underappreciated component of herpetological medicine, in part because most captive reptiles either do not survive to adulthood or have life spans shortened by inappropriate husbandry. This situation is in stark contrast to cardiology in domestic mammals, where much of the work related to primary cardiac disease can be tied to geriatric animals. As herpetoculture techniques improve and reptiles live longer, a similar interest may develop in herpetological medicine. For now, the primary relevance of clinical reptile cardiology is related to the impact of anesthetics and therapeutics on the circulatory system, with a minor component associated with the less common primary cardiac diseases.

CLINICAL ANATOMY AND PHYSIOLOGY

The circulatory system of reptiles has many basic similarities with the higher vertebrates (birds and mammals), including a multi-chambered heart, an arterial system that carries oxygenated blood through the body, a venous system that returns de-oxygenated blood to the heart, and a lymphatics system (without lymph nodes). There are, however, a number of differences that are of clinical importance.

The reptilian heart can be divided into two classifications: three-chambered or four-chambered. Some individuals consider the sinus venosus a fourth chamber in lower vertebrates and thus consider all reptiles to have four-chambered hearts.[2] The author prefers using the three- or four-chambered scheme, because the sinus venosus is both macroscopically and microscopically different from the standard atrial or ventricular chambers. In this article, the three- and four-chambered classifications are used.

Department of Veterinary Clinical Medicine, University of Illinois, College of Veterinary Medicine, 1008 W Hazelwood drive, Urbana, IL 61802, USA
E-mail address: mmitch@uiuc.edu

Vet Clin Exot Anim 12 (2009) 65–79
doi:10.1016/j.cvex.2008.10.001
1094-9194/08/$ – see front matter © 2009 Elsevier Inc. All rights reserved.

The three-chambered heart is common in the squamates (snakes and lizards) and chelonians, whereas the four-chambered heart is found in the crocodilians. The primary difference between the three- and four-chambered systems is the division of the ventricle. In crocodilians, a complete interventricular septum is found, whereas in squamates and chelonians the septum is incomplete. Although this incomplete septum does allow some blood mixing, the amount is minimized via contractions of the heart. In some species of chelonians the interventicular septal opening is small, resulting in what appears to be two separate ventricular chambers.

The location of the heart within the coelomic cavity varies among reptiles. In snakes, the heart is located at a distance approximately one third to one fourth of the body length from the head, although in certain aquatic species (*Nerodia* spp.) the heart can be in the proximal 15% to 20% of the body. In most cases, the snake heart can be located by placing the animal in dorsal recumbency and watching for the movement of the ventral scales (**Fig. 1**). The chelonian heart is located in the cranial coelomic cavity. In most species, it is located dorsal to the humeral and thoracic plastron scutes (**Fig. 2**). Of course, direct visualization of the beating heart is not possible in chelonians. The location of the lizard heart can vary among species. In agamids (eg, bearded dragons, *Pogona vitticeps*) and iguanids (eg, green iguanas, *Iguana iguana*), the heart is located at the level of the pectoral girdle (**Fig. 3**). By abducting the forelimb, it may be possible to see the heart beating through the axillary region. The location of the heart in monitor lizards (*Varanus* spp.) is more caudal (approximately one third to one fourth of the body length from the head) than that described for agamids and iguanids. The location of the crocodilian heart is similar to that described for monitor lizards.

The circulation of blood through the heart of squamates and chelonians is slightly modified from the model found in the four-chambered hearts of mammals and birds. Blood returning from the body drains through the precaval, postcaval, and hepatic veins into the sinus venosus. The sinus venosus is a muscular structure located on the dorsal surface of the right atrium that some authors consider to be a unique chamber.[2] During atrial diastole, blood from the sinus venosus is pumped into the right atrium. Atrial systole then directs the deoxygenated blood into the cavum venosum of the ventricle. This compartment of the ventricle, which is analogous to the right ventricular chamber of birds and mammals, is separated from the cavum arteriosum, or the "left ventricle," by the interventricular septum. Blood mixing between the

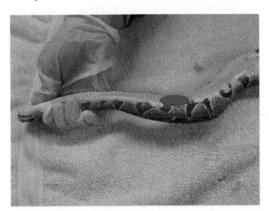

Fig. 1. The snake heart is located in the cranial fourth of the animal. The heart can be visualized most easily by placing the animal in dorsal recumbency and looking for the movement of ventral scales.

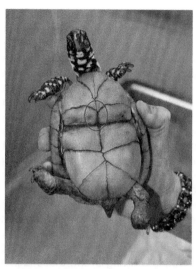

Fig. 2. The chelonian heart is located dorsal to the humeral the thoracic plastron scutes.

compartments is minimized by the occlusion of the canal by the atrioventricular valves, a series of muscular ridges in the ventricle, and the timing of the ventricular contractions.[3] Blood mixing does not occur in the crocodilian heart because the interventricular septum is complete. Deoxygenated blood leaving the right side of the heart is carried to the lungs via the pulmonary artery. The majority of the cardiac output (60%) is directed to the pulmonary circulation.[3] Oxygenated blood returns to the left atrium via the pulmonary vein. During atrial systole, the blood is pumped into the cavum arteriosum. Ventricular systole then directs the blood into the systemic circulation via the aorta.

Heart rates in reptiles are lower than those seen in avian and mammalian patients of similar size. This finding should not be surprising, because reptiles have lower metabolic rates than either birds or mammals.[4,5] In addition to differences based on metabolic rate, the environmental temperature, oxygen saturation levels in the blood, respiratory ventilation, postural stress, hemodynamic equilibrium, and body sensory stimuli can affect heart rate in reptiles.[6,7]

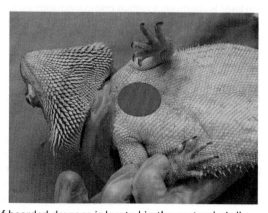

Fig. 3. The heart of bearded dragons is located in the pectoral girdle.

Reptiles are ectotherms and depend on their environmental temperature to regulate their core body temperature. Reptiles have adopted a number of behaviors to maximize their ability to increase or decrease their body temperature. Basking is a common behavior by which reptiles increase their core body temperature. During times of basking, reptiles increase their body temperature by increasing their heart rate. Vasodilation of the peripheral circulation during basking also increases body temperature. Reptiles exposed to excessive temperatures can develop life-threatening hyperthermia. To reduce body temperature, reptiles seek shelter, decrease their heart rate, and vasoconstrict their peripheral circulation. A less-than-optimal environmental temperature is a common cause for a reduced heart rate in a reptile during a physical examination or anesthetic event. It is important to optimize the environmental temperature of these animals during these procedures to avoid misclassifying an animal's true physiologic status.

Diving is a common behavior in aquatic reptiles. During periods of breath holding, pulmonary resistance increases to the point that blood flow to the lungs is reduced. To compensate, most reptiles reduce their heart rate and slow their metabolic rate. Crocodilians have developed a unique set of anatomic structures to accommodate them while under water. During a diving event, these animals close the glottis and hold their breath. Breath holding increases pulmonary tension, reducing blood flow from the pulmonary artery into the lungs and increasing the central pressure. To prevent this increased tension from serving as an obstacle to the blood flow to the systemic circulation, blood is shunted through the foramen of Pannizi into the left aorta and into the systemic circulation. This shunting allows the animals to remain under water until the oxygen levels are depleted to levels that are life threatening, at which time they must surface to take a breath. Non-crocodilian reptiles can shunt the blood within the heart to obtain the same effect. Persons working with these animals should consider this unique behavior when performing anesthetic procedures.

Blood pressure levels in reptiles are lower than those reported for higher vertebrates; however, there are exceptions for some species that have adapted their cardiopulmonary physiology to meet the demands of their hunting and reproductive needs.[8,9] The family Varanidae represents a small group of carnivorous lizards. To adapt to an active predatory lifestyle, these animals maintain blood pressure levels higher than those reported for other reptiles.[8] In addition to an elevated blood pressure, these animals are capable of maintaining ventricle pressure separation. Studies evaluating snakes, which also are carnivorous, found that most species did not maintain blood pressure levels comparable to the varanids.[8,9] An exception is the Burmese python (*Python molurus*).[9] This sit-and-wait predator is relatively inactive compared with varanids; therefore the relatively increased blood pressure measured in this species of snake may be associated with digestive or reproductive strategies and activity levels.[9]

The oxygen-carrying capacity of erythrocytes (hemoglobin) in reptiles can be affected by a number of different factors. During periods of voluntary apnea, reptiles can switch from aerobic to anaerobic glycolysis. The anaerobic cycle leads to the development of acidemia that severely reduces hemoglobin's carrying capacity for oxygen.

The vasculature of reptiles is similar to the model found in other higher vertebrates and includes arterial, venous, and lymphatic components. There are, however, some obvious differences in the reptilian circulatory system, such as the loss of the peripheral system associated with appendages in snakes. Snakes have developed interesting alterations in their vasculature to enable them to adapt to an apodan lifestyle. The vertebral venous plexus is a collection of spinal vessels surrounding the vertebral canal that allow blood to be shunted during times where blood flow might be compromised.[10]

One of the most controversial components of the reptile circulatory system is the renal portal system. Most veterinarians have been taught to avoid injecting therapeutic agents into the rear legs or tail of a reptile because of the risk of inducing renal disease. Much of this teaching originated from the first antibiotic pharmacokinetic studies in reptiles, in which injections of gentamicin were associated with renal disease.[11,12] More recent work suggests that the risk of nephrotoxicosis associated with injections in the caudal extremities may not pose as great a risk as once thought.[13,14] Research in red-eared slider turtles (*Trachemys scripta elegans*) suggests that the renal portal system is important during times of water deprivation.[13] Animals that are dehydrated can shunt blood through the renal portal system to perfuse the kidneys. The system is proposed to be associated with valves in the abdominal vein that have the ability to redirect blood through the iliac vessels and into the kidneys. Clinical pharmacokinetic research in snakes also suggests that the risk of renal complications may be low.[14] In carpet pythons (*Morelia spilota*), there was no significant difference in the distribution of a 200-mg/kg intramuscular injection of carbenicillin in the epaxial muscles in the cranial or caudal portion of the body. Renal impairment was not found to be a problem in any of the snakes. It is important to note that carbenicillin is not considered a nephrotoxic compound, and that the snakes were hydrated. Additional research is needed to determine the clinical importance of injection site in reptiles.

HISTORY AND PHYSICAL EXAMINATION CONSIDERATIONS

A thorough history can go far in directing a clinician who has a reptile patient with cardiovascular disease. Knowledge of the animal's signalment is important. Juvenile animals presenting with cardiovascular disease often have congenital anomalies or develop the disease secondary to inappropriate husbandry (eg, chronic low environmental temperature). Geriatric reptiles develop cardiovascular disease for the same reasons as mammals: over time, body systems tend to fail, worsen, or develop a problem. In green iguanas, for example, atherosclerosis sometimes is seen as a post-mortem finding in older animals and, as in humans, probably is related to diet, among other factors.

Inappropriate husbandry conditions, especially inadequate temperature and humidity, can be used to indicate the condition of a patient. Reptiles housed under low environmental temperatures may be more predisposed to chronic bradycardia, depressed respiratory ventilation, and a low metabolic rate. Low environmental humidity and limited access to drinking water or an inappropriate water delivery system may lead to chronic dehydration, which also can affect the cardiovascular system negatively. When requesting historical data for a patient, it is important to assess fully the environment and diet of the patient, because these factors can have an important impact on the cause and/or development of disease.

A reptile physical examination should be thorough and consistent. An understanding of an animal's activity and behavior patterns is important for characterizing normal versus abnormal behavior. For example, bearded dragons are naturally active, alert animals and during a physical examination should hold their head up, lick/taste the ground, and, in general, be inquisitive. If a dragon is lethargic, depressed, and exercise intolerant, these abnormal activities should be noted, and this information should be considered while working toward a final diagnosis.

Cardiovascular disease in reptiles may be manifested as a range of nonspecific clinical signs. Although it is natural to focus on cardiac function when considering cardiovascular disease, it also is important to consider the rest of the system. Ascites, peripheral edema, and organomegaly may be indicators of cardiovascular compromise. A final diagnosis can be made only through a thorough diagnostic work-up.

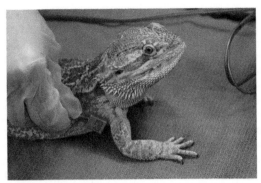

Fig. 4. To hear the heart sounds of a lizard with a heart located in the pectoral girdle, place the probe in the axillary region and direct it medially.

The cardiovascular system should be evaluated as a part of every routine examination. In mammals this evaluation is done by auscultating the animal, palpating for pulses (eg, femoral), and measuring indirect blood pressure. In many reptiles, these measurements may be difficult to collect. Auscultating reptiles has become a lost art. It is common for veterinarians to skip auscultating a reptile because they believe the practice is unrewarding. To the author, auscultating is always rewarding. Whether one can hear something or not is information that can be applied to the management of a case. When auscultating a reptile, it may be helpful to place a damp cloth over the auscultation field to minimize friction between the bell housing and scales. When the heart cannot be auscultated with a stethoscope, the author prefers to use a crystal ultrasonic Doppler probe. The Doppler probe provides an audible sound signal that enables the veterinarian to measure heart rate and assess heart sounds. In snakes, the Doppler probe can be placed directly over the heart. In lizards the probe can be placed in the axillary region and directed medially (**Fig. 4**). Because the varanid heart is located more caudally in the coelomic cavity, the probe should be placed over the lateral body wall at a distance of approximately one fourth of the body length from the head. For chelonians the probe can be placed between the base of the neck and forelimb and directed caudomedially (**Fig. 5**). A Doppler probe also can be used to assess blood pressure in reptiles, although in most cases it is not sensitive enough to obtain a reading that can be heard.

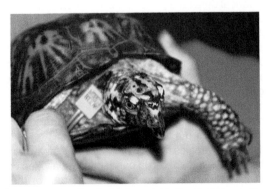

Fig. 5. To hear the heart sounds of a chelonian, place the Doppler probe at the base of the neck and direct it caudomedially.

DIAGNOSTIC TEST CONSIDERATIONS
ECG

The ECG is an underutilized diagnostic tool in reptile medicine. The primary reasons for its limited use are related to a limited amount of reference material to assist with interpretation and the limited degree of sensitivity associated with the available equipment.

When performing ECGs in reptiles, it is important to consider the physiologic status of the animal. Because heart and respiratory rates are linked to environmental temperature, it should be expected that ECGs will vary between and within species and even individual reptiles based on the environmental temperature at which the procedure is conducted. To maximize the value of the ECG, it always should be performed on an animal held in its optimal temperature range. This factor is especially important when performing serial ECGs on the same animal for comparison. An ECG can be collected on alert reptiles, although the author prefers to perform them under anesthesia to obtain the best recordings for interpretation. Reptile ECGs are naturally more difficult to interpret because of the low wave amplitudes of the different complexes, and minimizing the movements of the animal can improve the recording. For reptiles with limbs (eg, crocodilians, chelonians, lizards, tuataras), electrodes can be placed on the forelimbs and rear leg (down side), as is done with mammals (**Fig. 6**). In some cases the sensitivity of the ECG may be limited when using the legs, and placement of the cranial electrodes on the right and left lateral base of the neck may improve the recording. For snakes, cranial electrodes (**Fig. 7**) can be placed (1) two heart-lengths cranial to the heart (one on each lateral body wall) with a distal electrode placed caudal to the heart (60%–75% of the distance from the head) or (2) on the lateral body wall at the level of the heart, with a distal electrode placed as described previously. Electrodes can be attached using adhesive pads, direct placement of alligator clips, or by inserting hypodermic needles into the subcutaneous space and attaching the alligator clips directly to the needles. The author prefers to use adhesive pads for alert animals and the needle approach for anesthetized animals.

The reptile ECG has the same basic wave complexes seen in mammals and birds: P, QRS, and T. A fourth wave, the SV wave, may be seen in some species and represents the depolarization of the sinus venosus. When present, the SV wave is found before the P wave. A major difference in ECGs of reptiles and higher vertebrates is the amplitude of the wave complexes. For most reptiles, when the same sensitivity range

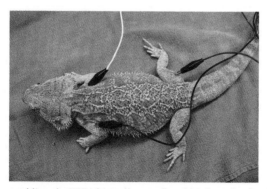

Fig. 6. In chelonians and lizards, ECG electrodes can be placed on the forelimbs and rear leg or body wall.

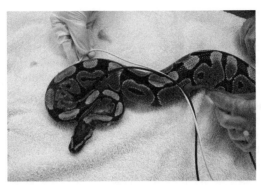

Fig. 7. In snakes, ECG electrodes can be placed cranial to the heart or at the level of the heart. The best technique often is decided on a case-by-case basis while reviewing the recordings.

is used, the amplitude of the complexes is much smaller than those found with mammals, resulting in an increased degree of difficulty with interpretation.

The general interpretation of a reptile ECG is as follows: (1) the SV wave signifies sinal contraction; (2) the P wave signifies atrial contraction; (3) the R wave signifies ventricular contraction; and (4) the T wave signifies ventricular depolarization. Findings can range widely when evaluating ECGs in reptiles. In red-ear slider turtles, depolarization is prolonged, with QT intervals averaging 1.4 seconds and mean RR intervals of 2.4 seconds.[15] The TP interval represents approximately one fourth of the cardiac cycle. The reptile ECG should not be considered a reference standard for a cardiologic examination in a reptile but instead as an important component of a cardiac diagnostic work-up. For example, Rishniw and Carmel[16] found that an ECG could be used with other diagnostic tools to confirm a diagnosis of atrioventricular valve insufficiency and congestive heart failure in a Carpet python. The ECG showed tall, wide QRS complexes.

There is limited reference material for interpreting ECGs in reptiles; therefore veterinarians should consider developing their own reference material. By performing ECGs in clinically healthy animals at the appropriate environmental temperature, it is possible to develop a set of reference values for the species most commonly presented to a practice.

Pulse Oximetry

Pulse oximetry was developed for mammals as a method of measuring oxygen saturation levels. One of the concerns with using this tool on reptiles was whether it could be validated. In green iguanas, absorbencies for oxyhemoglobin and deoxyhemoglobin were in agreement with those for mammals, suggesting it could be used in these animals.[17]

The probes provided by pulse oximeter manufacturers may have limited value in reptiles. The probes that seem to provide the most information are the esophageal and rectal probes. It was assumed that placement against the carotid or aorta would provide clinically relevant data, but placement of a probe against the carotid complex provided inconsistent results in green iguanas.[18] Pulse oximetry should be considered an auxiliary method for evaluating a reptile patient, with a primary function of providing insight into oxygen saturation trends for reptiles. The author considers Pa_{O_2} levels consistently above 90% acceptable, whereas levels that are consistently low (< 85%) should be re-evaluated using other diagnostic tools (eg, blood gas measurements).

Diagnostic Imaging

Survey radiographs

Survey radiographs remain an important component of a cardiac work-up. These diagnostic images enable the veterinarian to assess cardiac, pulmonary, vascular, and visceral structures of their patients. Heart size can be estimated in snakes and crocodilians. Comparing survey films from animals with clinical disease and those without disease may be helpful in characterizing the extent of disease. The heart of a lizard generally is not easy to visualize, because it is surrounded by the bony pectoral girdle. Varanids are an exception, because their hearts are located more caudally in the coelomic cavity (**Fig. 8**). The heart size of chelonians also is difficult to appreciate because of the superimposed bones of the carapace and plastron. Because cardiac disease can lead to secondary involvement of other organs, it is important to assess the entire patient when pursuing a case with cardiovascular disease. Pulmonary edema, hepatomegaly (organomegaly) associated with congestive heart failure, and mineralization of the vessels can be seen radiographically.

Ultrasound

Although echocardiography is a standard diagnostic tool used to assess cardiac disease in mammals, its use in reptile medicine is limited. The underutilization of this diagnostic method probably is associated with the availability/expense of the equipment, the training level of available users, and the general comfort level of veterinarians working with this diagnostic tool. As with endoscopy, however, this situation is likely to change as this diagnostic tool becomes more common.

The primary benefits of ultrasound are that it is noninvasive, accurate, and can be done ante mortem.[19] This diagnostic modality enables veterinarians to evaluate cardiac motion and function, heart valve function, cardiomegaly, pericardial effusion, structural deficits, and cardiac masses.[20] Color Doppler echocardiography also can be used to assess blood flow through and around the heart. This information is especially helpful when assessing anomalies associated with chamber filling, valvular defects, and the great vessels.

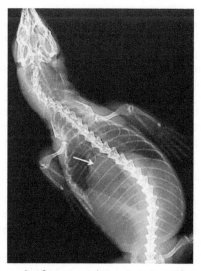

Fig. 8. Dorsoventral radiograph of a savannah monitor. Note the caudal positioning of the heart (*arrow*).

Probe size is an important consideration for ultrasonography. Because of the relative limited tissue depth of reptiles, higher-frequency (10–12 mHz) probes are preferred. These probes provide greater detail when evaluating tissues depths of 1 to 4 cm.

Snake hearts can be imaged by ultrasound by placing the probe directly over the ventral scales overlying the heart. In lizards, the probe can be placed in the axillary region and directed medially. For varanids and crocodilians, the probe should be placed more caudally on the lateral body wall. Because of the position of the ribs, there may be some bony interference. Approaches to the chelonian heart are limited to the cervicobrachial region. The probe should be placed between the neck and forelimb and directed caudomedially. It is important to use an appropriate amount of gel on the probe/animal to improve the resolution of an ultrasound image. If insufficient gel is used, it is possible that the scales may cause image interference. An ultrasound can also be performed with a reptile in a water bath.

Advanced imaging

CT and MRI are advanced diagnostic imaging methods that can be used to assess cardiac disease in reptiles. These imaging modalities are especially useful in chelonians, in which the presence of the shell limits the value of survey radiographs. The advantages of using CT are that the scan times are relatively short, visceral detail is excellent, and inhalant anesthesia can be used to complete the procedure. MRI also can provide high-detail images but may require more time to collect the images and the use of injectable anesthesia. Because CT is less expensive, it generally is done more frequently than MRI. The primary limitations associated with these diagnostic tools are the expense of the procedures and the availability of these imaging modalities to the general practitioner.

Plasma Biochemistry Testing

Plasma biochemistry data can be collected to evaluate the physiologic status of a reptile patient. Alterations in protein levels (eg, albumin) may help assess the hydration status of a patient and confirm a cause of edema. It is common to see hypoalbuminemia in reptiles presenting with peripheral edema, ascites, and anasarca. Creatine kinase is an enzyme that is released from damaged muscle cells, including skeletal, smooth, and cardiac muscle. In green iguanas, levels of this enzyme are highly correlated to cardiac muscle.[21] Aspartate aminotransferase also is found in cardiac muscle cells of reptiles and may be used with creatine kinase levels to assess cardiac disease. Alterations in electrolytes may result in cardiovascular disease. Because cardiac function can be altered by fluctuations in the minerals (eg, calcium, phosphorus) and electrolytes (eg, potassium, sodium), it is important to evaluate these levels also. Hyperuricemia can lead to visceral gout, and the heart is an organ in which gout tophi may be deposited. The clinical relevance of cholesterol levels in reptiles is not well understood but may be important when considering heart disease in reptiles.

CARDIOVASCULAR DISEASE CONSIDERATIONS

Cardiovascular disease in reptiles generally is considered an uncommon finding in captive animals; however, no large-scale, cross-sectional studies have been performed to determine the prevalence of cardiovascular disease in reptiles. Reptiles with cardiac disease often present with nonspecific clinical signs, including depression, lethargy, and weakness. It is possible that cardiovascular disease is more common than is generally accepted and that the current belief results from limited clinical and diagnostic experience. For this reason, it is important that veterinarians pursue a thorough history, physical examination, and diagnostic work-up when managing cardiovascular disease in a reptile case.

Congenital Disease

Developmental anomalies are common in captive reptiles and can include major problems such as the incomplete development of an embryo (eg, monsters) to less life-threatening anomalies such as incomplete closure of the umbilicus. The author has had a hatchling Brazilian rainbow boa (*Epicrates cenchria*) presented with incomplete migration and development of the viscera. In this animal, the heart was located just cranial to the mid-point of the snake, never migrating to its more natural position in the cranial one fourth of the snake. In this particular animal the ventral body wall never closed, and the major vital organs, including the heart, were visible. Closure of the ventral body wall was attempted, with the hope that continued development post-hatching might resolve the incomplete migration of the viscera; however, the animal never attempted to eat, was lethargic, and was euthanized 2 weeks after presentation. Incomplete development of specific cardiac structures also has been described.[3] A neonatal boa constrictor (*Boa constrictor*) presented for a swelling at the level of the heart. The animal was found to be bradycardic, to have an increased P-R interval, and to have a decreased Q-T interval compared with a clutch mate. Echocardiography suggested incomplete closure of the atrioventricular valves, and after the snake was euthanized, a post-mortem examination confirmed the incomplete development of the valves. Captive breeding is common practice, and congenital anomalies may be more common than expected. Some animals probably complete development of less vital anomalies post-hatchling, whereas others succumb because of the incomplete development of vital structures.

Nutrition-Related Disease

A reptile's heart rate can be affected by alterations in fluid balance. Hypoalbuminemia is a common finding in reptiles provided a less-than-optimal diet and/or with primary liver disease. Animals with hypoalbuminemia can present with edema, ascites, or anasarca as a result of fluid loss from the vascular space. To compensate for the fluid loss, the reptile's heart rate increases. It is important to correct the hypoalbuminemia and reduce oncotic pressure quickly in these patients. The use of liver-sparing compounds (eg, lactulose) and plasma expanders (eg, hetastarch) may be helpful.

Alterations in electrolytes also can have varying effects on a reptile's heart rate. Potassium is an essential electrolyte that is obtained through the diet. Animals provided less-than-optimal diets may develop hypokalemia. To compensate for the hypokalemia, potassium is released from the intracellular space to the extracellular space to ensure that potassium is available for vital functions, such as maintaining cell membrane potential and transmission of action potentials in nerve cells. Once the animal is provided glucose, however, the potassium moves back into the intracellular space. Affected animals can develop life-threatening arrhythmias. Similar findings can occur with animals that are hyperkalemic. Primary hyperkalemia generally is associated with renal disease. Animals that are hypokalemic should be provided potassium intravenously with their fluids and have their diet corrected. Hyperkalemic reptiles should be diuresed with fluids to maximize renal function. Bicarbonate can be given to counter metabolic acidosis. When arrhythmias are diagnosed, calcium may be used intravenously to counter myocardial excitability.

Dystrophic mineralization of the great vessels is a common finding in captive reptiles. A case of a ruptured aorta associated with mineralization of the aorta has been reported in a Chinese water dragon (*Physignathus concincinus*).[3] The animal previously had been diagnosed as having secondary nutritional hyperparathyroidism and a mandibular abscess. A post-mortem examination was done on the animal, because it died acutely, and mineralization was found in both the tunica interna and muscularis. The pathogenesis associated with this disease is not fully understood; however, it is thought that vitamin D may play a role.[22] In the past, vitamin D toxicity was considered to be the primary cause of dystrophic mineralization; however, more recent work suggests that these changes may be attributed to hypovitaminosis D. In humans, vascular calcification is associated with cardiovascular mortality.[23]

It always is important to review the diets of captive reptiles during the collection of the history. Obvious deficiencies should be addressed immediately. Less obvious deficiencies, such as the trace elements, may be more difficult to correct. Diversifying the diet of herbivores and omnivores and providing quality prey items to carnivores should minimize the likelihood of these problems. The provision of UVB radiation also is recommended. Historically, full-spectrum lighting was recommended for lizards, especially diurnal herbivorous species (eg, green iguana). Recent research in red-ear slider turtles and corn snakes (*Elaphe guttata*) suggests that these animals maintain higher 25-hydroxyvitamin D levels when provided appropriate lighting and that all diurnal reptile species may benefit from full-spectrum lighting to optimize calcium homeostasis.[24,25]

Secondary nutritional hyperparathyroidism was one of the most common disease presentations of reptiles during the past 2 decades. Fortunately, through better husbandry practices, this disease is not as common, although it still occurs with some frequency in herbivorous and insectivorous reptiles. Animals affected by this disease may present with weakness, lethargy, depression, muscle fasiculations, and seizures. Chronic renal failure in reptiles (eg, green iguanas) also can have a similar clinical presentation. In either case, affected reptiles may experience drastic fluctuations in calcium levels, resulting in the clinical signs described previously. Although the skeletal muscle changes are obvious, the cardiac changes may not be. Once the animal is stabilized, an ECG should be performed to evaluate cardiac function. These cases should be considered emergencies and treated accordingly.

Infectious Diseases

Infectious diseases have been associated with cardiovascular disease in reptiles. Most of the reports are attributed to bacterial infections. Because Gram-negative bacteria can be isolated from the blood of reptiles, thromboembolic disease of bacterial origin may be more common than currently thought. *Salmonella, Arizona*, and *Corynebacterium* sp. have been isolated from a Burmese python with endocarditis.[20] Chlamydiosis also has been associated with myocarditis in snakes.[26]

Viruses currently are not recognized as important pathogens associated with cardiovascular disease but should be considered. Parvovirus has been identified in juvenile bearded dragons with concurrent adenovirus infection.[27] In mammals, parvovirus has a predilection for cardiac muscle. The same may be true for reptiles, and additional research is needed to determine if a link exists.

Parasites

Filarid nematodes are a common finding in wild-caught reptiles. These parasites may be associated with the subcutaneous space, coelomic cavity, or cardiovascular system. Female filarids can release large numbers of larvae into the bloodstream, where they are taken up by blood-sucking vectors during feeding. The arthropods serve as a primary vector of these parasites. Affected animals generally are asymptomatic, although adult organisms may be seen occasionally in the subcutaneous tissues or intraocular chamber. Diagnosis can be made from a direct blood smear. Treatment may require surgical removal of the adult nematode. Removing reptiles from the wild, and thus eliminating exposure to the vector, also should break the life cycle. For patent infections, ivermectin (0.2 mg/kg once every 10 days for three treatments) is recommended, but this agent must not be used in chelonians. Anti-inflammatory agents also should be given to limit the potential formation of thromboemboli that may occur with the death of the nematodes.

Trematodes are parasites that typically are noted only in wild-caught reptiles as incidental findings at necropsy. One group of these parasites, the digenetic spirorchid trematodes, is associated with the cardiovascular system and can cause clinical disease. Spirorchid flukes are reported most often in aquatic chelonians. The life cycle of these parasites involves a gastropod intermediate host; therefore, the life cycle can be broken in captivity with the removal of the gastropods from the system. Adult flukes can be found in the heart and great vessels. Eggs are released and become lodged in peripheral vessels. Severe infestations can lead to mural endocarditis, arteritis, and thromboemboli formation. Diagnosis can be difficult, although an ELISA exists for the detection of antibodies in the green sea turtle (*Chelonia mydas*).[28] A direct blood smear also may be used to diagnose an infestation, if eggs are present. Praziquantel typically is recommended for the treatment of trematodes, although the efficacy of the drug against most trematodes is not known.[29]

Traumatic Injuries

Animals presenting after a traumatic injury, such as a chelonian with a crushing shell injury, or animals undergoing surgery that lose blood should be expected to have higher heart rates. In these situations, the reptile attempts to compensate for lower blood volume by increasing the heart rate. By increasing the heart rate, the reptile can ensure the delivery of oxygen to vital tissues. With acute blood loss, snakes compensate for the loss by shifting fluids from the intracellular space to the extracellular space.[6] In these cases, it is important to rehydrate these animals with appropriate fluids to expand the vascular space and allow the redistribution of fluids into the intracellular space. A combination of lactated Ringer's solution or saline and dextrose allows for the expansion of the vascular space and the intracellular spaces, respectively.

Miscellaneous Cardiovascular Diseases

Congestive heart failure

Congestive heart failure is a common finding in geriatric mammals. In reptiles, congestive heart failure is not considered common, perhaps because in captivity reptiles tend not to survive to the full extent of their lifespan. As husbandry methods improve, veterinarians may see more cases of congestive heart failure in their reptile patients. Congestive heart failure has been reported in a Burmese python.[20] The snake was found to have dilation of the right atrium and ventricular thickening. The snake also was found to have endocarditis. A mass obstructing the right atrioventricular valve was associated with obstructing blood flow into the heart.

Cardiomyopathy has been described in two species of snakes.[30,31] A mole king snake (*Lampropeltis calligaster rhombomaculata*) presented with lesions characterized by fibroblast proliferation and the replacement of myocardial fibrils with fibrocollagen.[30] A Deckert's rat snake (*Elaphe obsolete deckerti*) presented with necrosis of the myocardial fibers.[31] In both cases, the pathologic changes led to congestive heart failure. Therapy for such cases should follow the protocols outlined for mammals, realizing that success rate for these cases probably will be low. One of the problems encountered when trying to manage these cases is that drugs commonly used in mammals do not work in reptiles. For example, furosemide, commonly used to manage pulmonary edema in congestive heart failure, has little value in reptiles because it is a loop diuretic, and reptiles do not have a loop of Henle.

Aneurysms

Aneurysms have been described in snakes and lizards. An aortic aneurysm was reported in a Burmese python.[32] The animal presented with acute respiratory arrest after constricting its meal, a rabbit. At necropsy, a large, dissecting aortic aneurysm was found. Microscopically, there was separation of the muscular and intimal levels of the aorta. Aneurysms also have been described in bearded dragons. In these cases, the aneurysms are associated with the carotid vessels. Affected animals present with unilateral swelling in the cervical region. Performing a fine-needle aspiration of the area results in the collection of blood. The affected vessel can be ligated if the collateral circulation seems sufficient to maintain the animal.

SUMMARY

Reptile cardiology remains a specialty field in reptile medicine that receives little attention, but its importance will grow as veterinarians come to rely on anesthesia for more procedures and as reptiles live long enough to develop the types of cardiac disease seen in geriatric domestic mammals. Veterinarians should pursue cardiovascular cases in reptiles using the same methods described for mammals, while considering new methods of handling this unique group of animals. Veterinarians working with these cases should document their findings and share them with their colleagues to build an evidence-based foundation for reptile medicine.

REFERENCES

1. White FN. Circulation. In: Gans C, editor, Biology of the Reptilia, vol. 5. London: Academic Press Inc.; 1976. p. 273–334.
2. Girling SJ, Hynes B. Cardiovascular and haemopoietic systems. In: Girling SJ, Raiti P, editors. BSAVA manual of reptiles. 2nd edition. Quedgely (Gloucester): BSAVA; 2004. p. 243–60.
3. Kik MJL, Mitchell MA. Reptile cardiology: a review of anatomy and physiology, diagnostic approaches, and clinical disease. Se Avian Exotic Pet Med 2005;14(1): 52–60.
4. Dawson WR, Bartholomew GA. Relation of oxygen consumption to body weight, temperature, and temperature acclimation in lizards, *Uta stansburiana* and *Scleropus occidentalis*. Physiol Zool 1956;29:40–51.
5. Dawson WR, Bartholomew GA. Metabolic and cardiac responses to temperature in the lizard, *Dipsosaurus dorsalis*. Physiol Zool 1958;31:100–11.
6. Cabanac M, Bernieri C. Behavioral rise in body temperature and tachycardia by handling of a turtle (*Clemmys insculpta*). Behav Processes 2000;49:61–8.
7. Lillywhite HB, Zippel KC, Farrell AP. Resting and maximal heart rates in ectothermic vertebrates. Comp Biochem Physiol A 1999;124:369–82.
8. Porges SW, Riniolo TC, Bride T, et al. Heart rate and respiration in reptiles: contrast between a sit-and-wait predator and an intensive forager. Brain Cogn 2003;52:88–96.
9. Wang T, Altimiras J, Klein W, et al. Ventricular haemodynamics in *Python molurus*: separation of pulmonary and systemic pressures. J Exp Biol 2003;206:4241–5.
10. Zippel KC, Lillywhite HB, Mladinich RJ. New vascular system in reptiles: anatomy and postural hemodynamics of the vertebral venous plexus in snakes. J Morphol 2001;250:173–84.

11. Jacobson ER. Gentamicin related visceral gout in two boid snakes. Vet Med Small Anim Clin 1976;71:361–3.
12. Montali RJ, Bush M, Smeller JM. The pathology of nephrotoxicity of gentamicin in snakes. Vet Pathol 1979;16:108–11.
13. Holz PH. The reptilian renal portal system: influence on therapy. In: Fowler ME, Miller RE, editors. Zoo and wild animal medicine: current therapy 4. Philadelphia: WB Saunders; 1999. p. 249–51.
14. Holz PH, Burger JP, Pasloske K, et al. Effect of injection site on carbenicillin pharmacokinetics in the carpet python, *Morelia spilota*. J Herp Med Surg 2002;12(4): 12–5.
15. Holz RM, Holz P. Electrocardiography in anesthetized red-ear slider turtles (*Trachemys scripta elegans*). Res Vet Sci 1995;58:67–9.
16. Rishniw M, Carmel BP. Atrioventricular valve insufficiency and congestive heart failure in a carpet python. Aust Vet J 1999;77:580–3.
17. Diethelm G, Mader DR, Grosenbaugh DA, et al. Evaluating pulse oximetry in the green iguana (*Iguana iguana*). Proceedings of ARAV; 1998. p. 11–2.
18. Mosley CA, Dyson D, Smith DA. The cardiovascular dose-response effects of isoflurane alone and combined with butorphanol in the green iguana (*Iguana iguana*). Vet Anesth Analg 2004;31:64–72.
19. Snyder PS, Shaw NG, Heard DJ. Two-dimensional echocardiographic anatomy of the snake heart (*Python molurus bivittatus*). Vet Radiol Ultrasound 1999;40:66–7.
20. Jacobson ER, Homer B, Adams W. Endocarditis and congestive heart failure in a Burmese python (*Python molurus bivittatus*). J Zoo Wildl Med 1991;22:245–8.
21. Wagner RA, Wetzel R. Tissue and plasma enzyme activities in the common green iguana, *Iguana iguana*. Am J Vet Res 1999;60(2):201–3.
22. Allen ME, Oftedal OT. Nutrition in captivity. In: Jacobson ER, editor. Biology and husbandry of the green iguana. Malabar (FL): Krieger Publishing Company; 2003. p. 47–74.
23. Adragao T, Pires A, Lucas C, et al. A simple vascular calcification score predicts cardiovascular risk in haemodialysis patients. Nephrol Dial Transplant 2004;19:1480–8.
24. Acierno M, Mitchell MA, Roundtree M, et al. Effects of ultraviolet radiation on plasma 25-hydroxyvitamin D concentrations in corn snakes (*Elaphe guttata guttata*). Am J Vet Res 2008;69(2):294–7.
25. Acierno M, Mitchell MA, Roundtree M, et al. Evaluating the effect of ultraviolet B radiation on plasma 1.25-hydroxyvitamin D levels red-eared slider (*Trachemys scripta elegans*). Am J Vet Res 2006;67(12):2046–9.
26. Jacobson ER, Gaskin JM, Mansell J. Chlamydial infection in puff adders (*Bitis arietans*). J Zoo Wildl Med 1989;20:364–9.
27. Kim DY, Mitchell MA, Bauer R. An outbreak of adenoviral infection in inland bearded dragons (*Pogona vitticeps*) coinfected with Dependovirus and coccidial protozoa (*Isospora* sp.) J Vet Diagn Invest 2002;14:332–4.
28. Gordon A, Kelly WR, Cribb TH. Lesions caused by cardiovascular flukes (Digenea: Spirorchidae) in stranded green turtles (*Chelonia mydas*). Vet Pathol 1998;35:21–30.
29. Murray MJ. Cardiology and circulation. In: Mader D, editor. Reptile medicine and surgery. Philadelphia: WB Saunders; 1996. p. 95–104.
30. Barten SL. Cardiomyopathy in a king snake (*Lampropeltis calligaster rhombomaculata*). Vet Med Small Anim Clin 1980;75:125–9.
31. Jacobson ER, Seely JC, Novilla MN, et al. Heart failure associated with unusual hepatic inclusions in a Deckert's rat snake. J Wildl Dis 1980;15:75–81.
32. Rush EM, Donnelly TM, Walberg J. What's your diagnosis? Cardiopulmonary arrest in a Burmese python. Lab Anim 2001;30:24–7.

Cardiovascular Physiology and Diseases of Pet Birds

Michael Pees, DrMedVet, DECAMS*,
Maria-Elisabeth Krautwald-Junghanns, DrMedVet, DECAMS

KEYWORDS

• Bird • Heart • Physiology • Pathology • Diagnostics • Therapy

Even though most gross structures of the avian cardiovascular system are similar to those of mammals, some details are unique. The avian heart is a capable organ that meets the high demands during flight and in extreme situations. Whereas cardiac diseases are comparably rare in wild birds, in pet birds—especially parrots—they play a more important role. Based on technical and research progress, we can now diagnose and treat cardiac disease in the avian patient.

ANATOMY AND PHYSIOLOGY OF THE AVIAN CARDIOVASCULAR SYSTEM

The avian heart lies in the cranioventral part of the coelomic cavity, slightly to the right of midline and in close sternal contact. Because a diaphragm is lacking, the apex is surrounded by liver tissue. A fibrous pericardium encloses the heart and a small amount of pericardial fluid. The mass of the avian heart is approximately twice the mass of a mammal's heart of comparable size but varies depending on species, habitat, and way of life. As in mammals, the avian heart is four-chambered and provides systemic and pulmonary circulation to the body. Because the resistance to blood flow is significantly less in the pulmonary circulation, the right ventricle is thin-walled and lies in a sickle-moon shape around the thick-walled left ventricle. The left ventricle is cone-shaped and, unlike the right, extends to the apex of the heart. The outer shape is dominated by a nearly plain facies dorsocaudalis muscle facing the lung and a convex facies ventrocranialis muscle near the sternum (**Fig. 1**). The right aspect of the heart is slightly concave, and the left one is convex. These contours can be seen on radiographs (**Fig. 2**). The atria are thin-walled, and the right atrium is larger than the left one. In contrast to mammals, the atrioventricular opening of the left side is marked by a tricuspid valve, whereas between the right atrium and ventricle, there is a rectangular-shaped muscular atrioventricular valve unique to the avian heart. It is

Clinic for Birds and Reptiles, University of Leipzig, An den Tierkliniken 17, 04103 Leipzig, Germany
* Corresponding author.
E-mail address: pees@vmf.uni-leipzig.de (M. Pees).

Vet Clin Exot Anim 12 (2009) 81–97
doi:10.1016/j.cvex.2008.08.003
1094-9194/08/$ – see front matter © 2009 Elsevier Inc. All rights reserved.

vetexotic.theclinics.com

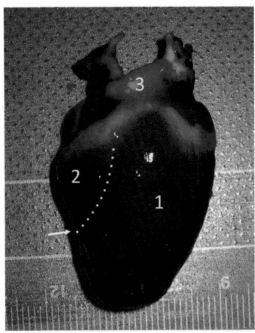

Fig. 1. Outer anatomy of a normal psittacine heart: the left ventricle (1) is prominent, whereas the right one (2) is small and does not reach the apex of the heart. An impression of the outer shape is visible (*arrow*) at the apex of the right ventricle (3, aorta/truncus brachiocephalicus).

assumed that this valve supports the complete emptying of the right ventricle. The aorta starts from the left ventricle with a tricuspid valve and turns slightly to the right side of the coelomic cavity. Immediately after the outflow of the coronary arteries, the aorta divides into the aorta descendens and two trunci brachiocephalici that supply the wings and head.[1]

Physiology of the avian heart is adjusted to high-performance demands. Birds have bigger stroke volumes, larger cardiac outputs, and the ability to increase the heart rate to 1000 beats per minute based on the species. This allows for high oxygen demand during flight. The small diameter of the cardiac muscle fibers (approximately one fifth of those of mammals) allows for rapid oxygen and energy distribution. The atria are considered to be a blood reservoir for ventricular filling rather than an important part of the hemodynamic process.[2]

As mammals, birds have a cardiac conduction system consisting of a sinuatrial node, an atrioventricular node, and Purkinje fibers. The sinuatrial node is the primary pacemaker, from which the electrical impulse moves to the atrioventricular node and by way of the atrioventricular bundle to the ventricles. An additional atrioventricular ring allows for fast depolarization of the ventricles. In contrast to mammals, the ventricular depolarization is not directed from the endocardium to the outer side of the heart but is rather diffuse, which might explain the negative QRS wave in birds.[3]

CARDIAC DISEASES IN BIRDS

In addition to individual case reports, two systematic postmortem studies exist on the pathology of the avian heart.[4,5] Both show a high incidence of cardiac alterations in pet

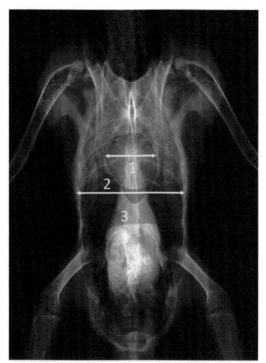

Fig. 2. Radiograph of a healthy scarlet macaw (*Ara macao*), ventrodorsal view. The size of the heart (1) can be set in relation to the width of the thorax (2). The liver lies next to the heart, surrounding the apex. The liver shadow (3) should be less wide than the heart shadow.

birds. In a study of 269 psittaciformes, congestive heart failure was found in 9.7% of all animals examined.[4] A total of 5.6% of these animals, more than 50% of birds with macroscopic heart lesions, probably died from primary heart disease. An additional study[5] found macroscopic changes of the heart or the great vessels in 36% of 107 psittaciformes. Pericardial effusion was found in 6% of these birds, serofibrinous coating on the pericardium in 15%, and hypertrophy or dilatation of the ventricular myocardium in 15% (**Fig. 3**). Other findings were petechial hemorrhage in the heart musculature and thrombotic valvular endocarditis. Within the wall of the aorta and the pulmonal artery, focal yellowish discoloration and hardening could be seen in 10% of these birds. In 99% of birds examined, at least low-grade histologic changes of the heart or the large vessels were found. The main histopathologic findings were inflammatory, mixed-cellular infiltrations of the myocardium (59.8%), focal coagulation (23.4%), and lipomatosis cordis (48.6%). In 13.1% of birds, atherosclerotic changes of the large vessels were found histologically. In conclusion, cardiac disease in pet birds plays a by far greater role than previously assumed, and examination of the heart should be included as part of routine physical examination and diagnostic testing in birds.

DIAGNOSTIC POSSIBILITIES

Despite considerable advances in diagnosing cardiac diseases in birds, there are still some complicating factors. The clinical signs and anamnestic data are nonspecific in

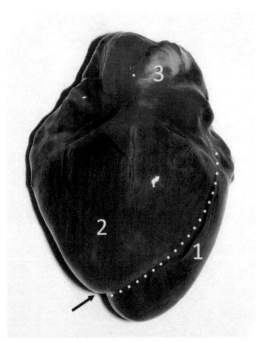

Fig. 3. Psittacine heart of a blue-fronted Amazon parrot (*Amazona aestiva*) that has right ventricular insufficiency. The right ventricle (2) is strongly dilated and nearly as large as the left one (2). The arrow indicates the apex of the right ventricle.

most cases, giving only a few hints about the cause of the circulatory problem. Additionally, heart disease is often a secondary problem (eg, after an infectious process); thus, symptoms of other organ alterations or diseases may overlay the clinical picture. Furthermore, the cardiovascular system is difficult to assess during clinical examination because the peripheral pulse is difficult to palpate and ausculta- tion is difficult to evaluate. Therefore, the diagnosis of the origin and extent of the disease process is mainly achieved using diagnostic techniques, such as electrocar- diography (ECG), radiography, and sonography. These methods may be complicated by the size of the patient, high heart rates, and the lack of reference values or diagnos- tic experience in avian species. Experience is especially limiting and frustrating because special cardiac diagnostics require profound expertise of the examiner. The diagnostic procedures that are discussed in this article include clinical examina- tion; radiography, including angiocardiography and CT; sonography, including Dopp- ler echocardiography; and ECG.

Clinical Examination

The clinical diagnosis of cardiovascular disease in live birds is difficult or even impos- sible in many cases. Clinical examination findings can provide an indication for further diagnostic measures, however.

Birds that have heart disease are normally presented to the veterinarian with a history of weakness and apathy. In some cases (especially in African gray parrots), cardiovas- cular insufficiency can be suspected based on a bluish discoloration of the periorbital skin, a sunken periorbital region (**Fig. 4**), or edema of the legs or wings, respectively.

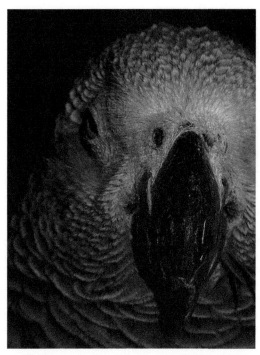

Fig. 4. African gray parrot (*Psittacus erithatus erithacus*) that has cardiovascular insufficiency. Note the sunken periorbital region and the bluish discoloration of the skin in this area.

Nonspecific symptoms, such as dyspnea and exercise intolerance, may also lead to the suspicion of cardiovascular disorders. In case of pericarditis within the context of acute visceral gout, plasma uric acid levels may be increased. Pericardial effusion may be found concurrently with profound dyspnea, weakness, and abdominal swelling. These clinical signs can also occur in cases of hepatic congestion and ascites, however. These clinical signs of myocardial insufficiency can also present as generalized weakness or as respiratory impairment. Alterations of the endocardium, particularly of the valves, are often seen after septicemia and may be accompanied by weakness or dyspnea, ascites, and a reduced general condition. Arteriosclerosis may occur more frequently in African gray parrots, macaws, and Amazon parrots older than 15 years of age. Age and nutritional deficiencies over many years and a lack of exercise may also predispose to the development of arteriosclerosis. Arteriosclerosis may not be diagnosed in early stages based on a lack of clinical signs. Unfortunately, in advanced stages, acute death may occur. Early clinical signs range from neurologic symptoms, including lameness, to lethargy. Later disease signs include vomiting or dyspnea, partially with rattling breathing, culminating in the development of ascites.

Radiographic Techniques

Standard plain radiography is a commonly performed imaging technique in avian medicine. The apex of the heart is overlaid by the liver, and these two organs form the shape of an hourglass in the ventrodorsal view. In this view, the aorta and other large vessels are projected in an oblique direction and may be seen as round radiodense structures at the base of the heart. In the lateral view, the brachiocephalic trunk,

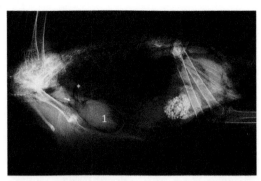

Fig. 5. Radiograph of a healthy sulfur-crested cockatoo (*Cacatua citrinocristata*), lateral view. In cockatoos, the apex of the heart (1) is well defined against the surrounding tissue. The aorta (*) and the trunci brachiocephalici (*arrow*) can also be assessed.

the aorta, and parts of the pulmonary arteries can be assessed. Normally, the radiographic examination is not undertaken specifically to look for cardiovascular disease. Radiographs often reveal information about alterations of the heart's size and shape by chance, however, and give an indication for an ultrasound examination (normal radiographs; see **Fig. 2; Fig. 5**). Furthermore, the radiograph may show secondary changes that may arise in other organs, such as increased radiodensity of the lungs, enlargement of the hepatic silhouette, or ascites in case of congestive heart failure. Alterations of heart size usually appear as an enlargement of the heart shadow. Ascites can mask the radiographic detail of the coelomic body cavity (**Fig. 6**). Cardiovascular disorders may also displace the air sac regions. Unfortunately, radiographic differentiation among the different causes for cardiac enlargement, such as dilatation, hypertrophy, pericardial effusion, granulomas, and tumors, is rarely possible. Alterations of the cardiac shape are attributable to several causes, such as dilation of one heart chamber.

Alterations of the large heart vessels (often visible as increased radiodensity) are marked by round shadows superimposed to the heart's silhouette in ventrodorsal projections. In the laterolateral projection, these vessels (eg, the aorta) appear as enlarged radiodense structures.[6]

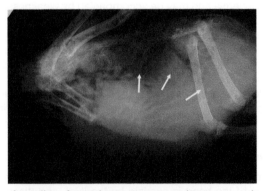

Fig. 6. Radiograph of a yellow-fronted Amazon parrot (*Amazona ochrocephala*) that has cardiac insufficiency, lateral view. The air sacs are displaced because of the increased heart and liver shadow (*arrows*). Because of ascites, detail recognition in the coelomic cavity is strongly reduced.

Advanced stages of arteriosclerosis can sometimes be seen as a combination of increased radiodensity and widening of the aorta and accompanying ventricular dilatation. Pericarditis may appear as cardiomegaly with an irregular cardiac silhouette. Pericardial effusion can occur secondary to congestion in other organs. Thus, radiography may demonstrate cardiac silhouette enlargement and organomegaly or ascites. In the case of myocarditis, the silhouette of the heart in the radiograph may be consolidated, which is seen as increased radiodensity.

Measurements of the length and width of the cardiac silhouette on radiographs have limitations. The superimposition of the apex of the heart and the liver in laterolateral and ventrodorsal projections or of the ventral parts of the heart and the sternum, respectively, in laterolateral projections often make measurements of cardiac silhouette length impractical. An exception occurs in cockatoos, in which the position of the surrounding cranial thoracic air sacs and air is a negative contrast medium in radiography and leads to good visualization of the heart's apex (see **Fig. 5**). Generally, the cardiac silhouette width is measured on ventrodorsal radiographs. For these measurements, exact positioning of the bird with correct superimposition of the keel and the spine is necessary. To assess the width of the cardiac silhouette, the measured value should relate to the thoracic width. Both measurements are performed at the maximum width of the cardiac silhouette (see **Fig. 2**). Alternately, the length of the sternum is used to assess cardiac size in relation to body size.[7] In medium-sized psittacines (approximately 200–500 g), the width of the cardiac shadow should be approximately 36% to 41% of the sternal length or 51% to 61% of the thoracic width, respectively.[7] In the Canada goose, the width of the cardiac silhouette should be 47% to 57% of the thoracic width.[8]

Indications for angiocardiography in birds are currently limited to the diagnosis of (congenital) vascular disorders and morphologic alterations of the heart not detectable by ECG and echocardiography. Contractility of the ventricles and the extent of the atria may be assessed, although there are no systematic studies on angiocardiographic investigations in birds (**Fig. 7**). Case reports about the use of angiocardiography exist on the diagnosis of aneurysm of the right coronary artery in a white cockatoo[9] and cardiomegaly in a whooper swan.[10] For angiocardiography, the avian patient must be anesthetized for intravenous injection of a non-ionic iodine contrast medium (iodine, 250 mg/mL, 2–4 mL/kg with an administration rate of approximately 1–2 mL/s). An image series of several images per second in dorsal or lateral recumbency should be obtained.

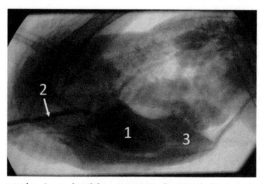

Fig. 7. Angiocardiography in a healthy common buzzard (*Buteo buteo*), lateral view. Contrast medium was given by way of the jugular vein (2) and is just floating into the heart chambers (1) (3, liver).

Although the use of CT for the diagnosis of vascular disorders is recommended in human medicine, visualization of the heart and its vessels is difficult because of movement of the organ. This problem is amplified in avian medicine. To reduce movement artifacts and have proper positioning, isoflurane anesthesia is necessary. Positioning is in dorsal recumbency, with slightly spread wings and with the hind limbs extended as far caudally as possible. A restraint plate, without metal screws to reduce the risk for artifacts, can be used for fixation. The examination can be done along the long axis (axial views) and the short axis (transversal views) of the bird. A slice thickness of 0.6 to 2 mm is used in most avian patients. In contrast to conventional radiography, in which only the cardiac silhouette may be examined, the chambers of the heart may be differentiated after application of contrast medium. Contrast medium is necessary because muscle and blood are of similar radiodensity, and thus may not be distinguishable on the native tomogram.

Indications for an examination by CT for diagnosis of cardiovascular disease in birds are rare. Little is known regarding the possibility of diagnosing vascular alterations as in human medicine (eg, infarction, abdominal aortic aneurysm) in birds, and reference values for assessment and densities are lacking. Advantages of CT may include diagnosis of alterations of the vessel walls (eg, calcinosis, atherosclerosis) and partial blockade of vessels as the result of thrombus. Neoplasms and granulomas or calcifications may also be seen.

Sonographic Techniques

Echocardiography is one of the most important imaging techniques for diagnosing cardiovascular disorders in birds. It enables the veterinarian to obtain information on the structure, size, and plane of motion of the avian heart. As a result of technical progress, suitable ultrasound machines are now readily available and affordable. Therefore, the number of practitioners with sonographic experience and special equipment increases from year to year.

Echocardiography demands certain equipment specifications for successful use in birds. The scanner should be a microcurved probe with a frequency of at least 7.5 MHz. These probes have a small coupling surface and can be coupled on the ventromedian approach directly behind the sternum. The frequency is necessary to visualize the small structures in the avian heart. For the examination, the ultrasound machine needs to achieve frame rates of 100 or higher, because birds can have extremely high heart rates. An additional color- and spectral-Doppler option is preferable. Finally, simultaneous ECG recording is recommended to allow measurements at definite stages of the heart cycle.

To determine normal and abnormal echocardiographic values in birds, it is important to have a standard protocol for the ultrasonographic examination.[11] Because the food-filled gastrointestinal tract might be interposed between the scanner and the heart (bone and gas block the passage of ultrasound waves), fasting birds before the sonographic examination is recommended. Fasting is unnecessary in severely diseased anorexic patients, however, or in those that have been fasted during transport to the veterinarian. In most patients, B-mode echocardiography can be performed without sedation or anesthesia. Only birds extremely sensitive to handling-induced stress should be anesthetized. Because of the bird's sensitivity for circulatory suppression, avian patients should be examined in a partially upright position. For this purpose, the bird is best held by the owner or an assistant or can be restrained on a suitable holding device. Because of the avian anatomy, sonographic approaches to the heart are limited. In psittacines and raptors, the ventromedian approach is routinely used. If necessary (not in parrots), some feathers are plucked and water-soluble acoustic gel is applied to the skin. The scanner is placed vertically on the midline of the abdomen, immediately caudal to the sternum with the beam plane directed craniodorsally. From this position, two longitudinal cross sections of the heart are found, the two-chamber view and the four-chamber view, which are produced by a 90° rotation of the scanner. The two-chamber view shows the left ventricle and the left atrium in addition to the left atrioventricular valve. Small parts of the right ventricle may also be seen. The four-chamber view shows both ventricles, the atrioventricular valve, and the aortic root with the aortic valve and parts of the atria (**Fig. 8**).[12,13] Because of anatomic differences in pigeons and some other bird species with a larger boneless space between last rib and pelvis, a parasternal approach may also be used. This approach allows several long-axis and short-axis views to be obtained.

For the assessment of the heart, the widest transverse and longitudinal diameter of the left and right ventricles should be measured in systole and diastole. Reference values have been established for psittaciformes,[12,13] birds of prey,[14] and pigeons (**Table 1**).[15] The calculated fractional shortening in healthy psittacines is approximately 23.1% ± 4.6%. In pigeons, a value of approximately 17% has to be considered physiologically normal. The calculated relation of the width to the length of the left ventricle is crucial for the assessment of ventricular dilatation and is relatively constant for some examined psittacine species (0.33 systolic, 0.40 diastolic).[13]

Altered cardiac wall thicknesses and decreased contractility can be assessed (**Figs. 9** and **10**) in addition to dilated vessels within the liver parenchyma, indicating congestion. Structural changes and dysfunction of the valves can also be demonstrated (in combination with color-Doppler echocardiography). In the authors' experience, ultrasonographic investigation may be of value for diagnosis of arteriosclerotic processes of the large vessels close to the heart, because they appear thickened and hyperechoic. This diagnosis is still most commonly done at necropsy, however. In pericarditis, the sonographic investigation demonstrates a consolidated density in the pericardium. Pericardial effusion can be visualized clearly as an anechoic structure between the myocardium and the pericardium around the heart (**Fig. 11**). In individual cases, a sonographically guided aspirate may be taken from the pericardium and examined cytologically or microbiologically.

Pulsed-wave spectral-Doppler echocardiography is the standard method for noninvasive blood flow velocity measurements. The ventromedian approach displays the

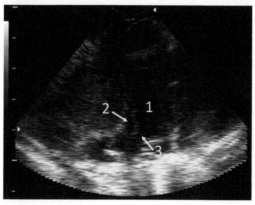

Fig. 8. Ultrasound examination in a blue-fronted Amazon parrot (*Amazona aestiva*), horizontal "four-chamber" view. The heart lies embedded in liver tissue, with a prominent left (1) and a small right (2) ventricle (3, aortic root).

Table 1
Echocardiographic parameters in selected avian species (given based on a ventromedian approach, mean value ± standard deviation)

Parameter	Psittacus e. erithacus[13]	Amazona spp[13]	Cacatua spp[13]	Diurnal Raptors[14]
Body mass (g)	493 ± 55	353 ± 42	426 ± 162	720 ± 197
Left ventricle				
Length systole (mm)	22.5 ± 1.9	21.1 ± 2.3	19.0 ± 1.3	14.7 ± 2.8
Length diastole (mm)	24.0 ± 1.9	22.1 ± 2.2	19.9 ± 1.6	16.4 ± 2.7
Width systole (mm)	6.8 ± 1.0	6.7 ± 1.2	6.4 ± 1.7	6.3 ± 1.1
Width diastole (mm)	8.6 ± 1.0	8.4 ± 1.0	8.3 ± 1.5	7.7 ± 1.2
Width fractional shortening (%)	22.6 ± 4.4	22.8 ± 4.2	25.6 ± 7.0	Not given
Right ventricle				
Length systole (mm)	9.2 ± 1.4	9.4 ± 1.8	10.3 ± 1.2	12.7 ± 2.7
Length diastole (mm)	11.5 ± 1.9	10.3 ± 1.3	11.3 ± 2.3	13.9 ± 2.5
Width systole (mm)	2.8 ± 0.9	3.1 ± 0.7	2.3 ± 0.0	2.1 ± 0.6
Width diastole (mm)	4.8 ± 1.1	5.2 ± 1.3	3.5 ± 0.5	2.5 ± 0.8
Width fractional shortening (%)	40.8 ± 11.9	34.1 ± 3.7	33.3 ± 10.3	Not given
Interventricular septum				
Thickness systole (mm)	2.9 ± 0.5	2.2 ± 0.1	1.9 ± 0.3	1.9 ± 0.6
Thickness diastole (mm)	2.5 ± 0.3	2.1 ± 0.4	1.7 ± 0.4	1.9 ± 0.5

heart along the long axis; therefore, measurements in the areas of the atrioventricular openings and the great vessels are easy to obtain (**Fig. 12**). Handling-induced stress significantly increases the intracardial blood flow velocity, whereas anesthesia decreases the velocity. Thus, Doppler echocardiography should be performed under anesthesia. Scientific studies of spectral-Doppler echocardiography in birds are

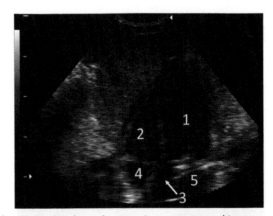

Fig. 9. Ultrasound examination in a vinaceus Amazon parrot (*Amazona vinacea*) that has decompensated cardiomyopathy, horizontal "four-chamber" view. The right ventricle (2) and the left one (1) are dilated, and the walls are thinned (3, aorta; 4, right ventricle; 5, right ventricle).

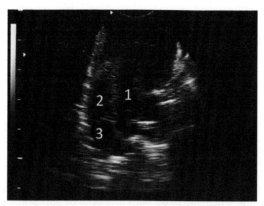

Fig. 10. Ultrasound examination in a yellow-fronted Amazon parrot (*Amazona ochrocephala*) that has hypertrophic cardiomyopathy of the right ventricle, vertical view. The right ventricle (2) is nearly as large as the left one (1). The walls are thickened (3, right atrium).

limited. Color-Doppler echocardiography has yet to be used in assessment of avian hearts, whereas pulsed-wave Doppler echocardiography has been applied in psittacines and raptors to detect diastolic inflow into the left and right ventricles in addition to systolic aortic outflow.[16–18] Blood flow within the pulmonal artery has not been examined, however. Selected reference values for velocities are given in **Table 2**.

Color-Doppler echocardiography (**Fig. 13**) can be used for the detection of valvular insufficiencies in birds. It is also helpful for the positioning of the Doppler gate for pulsed-wave Doppler analysis to estimate valvular insufficiency. Unfortunately, the use of the color-Doppler mode reduces the frame rate and the ability to demonstrate cardiac blood flow. Only case reports document the extent of use of color-Doppler echocardiography in birds.

Electrocardiography

Based on difficulties with the connection of the leads to the skin and stress-induced alterations, ECG is used less frequently in birds compared with mammals. It is a useful

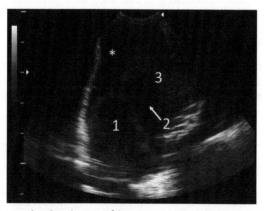

Fig. 11. Ultrasound examination in an African gray parrot (*Psittacus erithatus erithacus*), vertical view. The heart (1) lies in the fluid-filled pericardial cavity, and the pericardium (2) is visible. Ascites (*) is also present (3, liver).

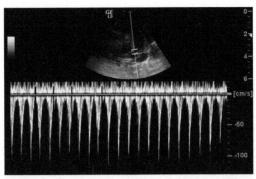

Fig. 12. Ultrasound examination in a healthy African gray parrot (*Psittacus erithatus eritha-cus*). The aortic outflow is demonstrated, with a velocity of approximately 100 cm/s.

technique for diagnosis and control of arrhythmias, conduction disorders, and detecting ventricular enlargement and metabolic disorders, however.[19] Further indications include monitoring cardiac function during anesthesia, triggering cardiac stages (eg, systole, diastole) while performing echocardiography, and monitoring the therapy of cardiac disease.

Anesthesia is recommended by some investigators to prevent stress-induced alterations, whereas others prefer recording the ECG in the awake bird, because anesthesia may also induce ECG alterations. Arrhythmias, second- and third-degree atrioventricular block, sinus arrest, T-wave depression, and atrial premature contraction have been described with isoflurane anesthesia.[20]

Six leads, as commonly performed in mammals, can be used, but a paper speed of at least 100 mm/s is necessary because of the high heart rates. Leads are attached on the right wing (RA), left wing (LA), and left limb (LL), and the right limb is connected to the ground.[21] Leads can be attached to the skin or the feathers using subcutaneous needles or alligator clips that are attached to the base of a feather with some ECG gel to provide the electrical connection to the skin.

The avian ECG is different from the mammalian ECG. A lead II ECG complex typical for a healthy bird is demonstrated in **Fig. 14**. ECG reference values exist for racing pigeons,[22] Amazon parrots, African gray parrots,[23] and some macaw species.[24]

THERAPEUTIC POSSIBILITIES

Therapy of cardiac disease in birds is still in its infancy. There are only few scientific studies about the use of cardiac drugs in birds, and only case reports exist for newer drugs. Nevertheless, these reports indicate the use of cardiac drugs for birds as for mammals.

Table 2			
Intracardial velocities in select avian species (anesthetized, mean value ± standard deviation)			
Parameter	*Amazona* spp[18]	*Falco* spp[16]	*Buteo buteo*[16]
Diastolic inflow left ventricle (m/s)	0.18 ± 0.03	0.21 ± 0.03	0.14 ± 0.01
Diastolic inflow right ventricle (m/s)	0.22 ± 0.05	0.21 ± 0.04	0.14 ± 0.02
Systolic outflow aortic root (m/s)	0.83 ± 0.08	0.95 ± 0.07	1.18 ± 0.05

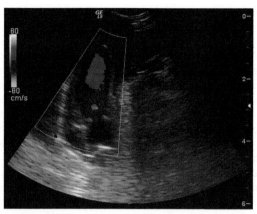

Fig. 13. Color-Doppler ultrasound examination in an African gray parrot (*Psittacus erithatus erithacus*). Filling of the left ventricle is demonstrated.

When treating birds with cardiac disease, note that most avian cardiac cases are high-grade alterations that are first diagnosed in some stage of decompensation. Accompanying symptoms, such as weakness, emaciation, ascites, and high-grade circulatory disturbances, are normally present and must also be addressed. All birds with cardiac problems should be considered as emergency cases with acute life-threatening illness.

Generally, three goals exist for therapy of cardiac diseases in birds: heart or circulatory medication, surgical removal of fluid (pericardiocentesis), and supportive or adjunctive therapy. In addition, therapy of the primary cause of disease (eg, aspergillosis) is necessary.

Cardiac or Circulatory Drugs

The use of heart glycosides has been studied in sparrows (*Passer domesticus*), budgerigars (*Melopsittacus undulatus*), and monk parakeets (*Myiopsitta monachus*).[25,26] The therapeutic margin in birds is small, and side effects mimic the symptoms that

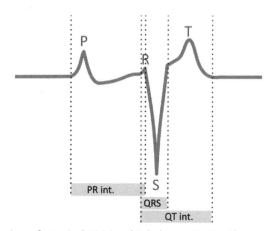

Fig. 14. Schematic view of a typical ECG in a bird, demonstrating the prominent RS-complex that represents ventricular depolarization.

indicate using these drugs (lethargy, anorexia, vomitus, and diarrhea). Additionally, a variable elimination time in different species may lead to accumulation of heart glycosides. In the authors' experience, heart glycosides are of use for emergency cases to stabilize birds. Long-term administration may be problematic, because controlling effect and plasma levels is difficult, and sudden death may occur. The authors recommend an initial dosage of digoxin at 20 to 50 µg/kg administered twice daily, with maintenance dosed carefully at 10 µg/kg administered twice daily.

Antiarrhythmics have been studied primarily in poultry. Before starting a therapy with antiarrhythmics, other causes for arrhythmias, such as potassium deficiency, must be excluded. The safety margin of these drugs is small, and the half-life is short. In turkeys, beta-blockers, such as oxprenolol (2 mg/kg administered orally once daily), have a protective effect against the development of atherosclerotic plaques.[27,28]

Angiotensin-converting enzyme (ACE) blockers are effective and safe drugs in pigeons and parrots. Clinically available drugs are captopril and enalapril. Because the half-life and efficacy of enalapril is greater than those of captopril, this drug is preferred for use in birds. Pigeons dosed at 10 mg/kg over 3 weeks showed no change in clinical and laboratory parameters. The recommended dosage in Amazon parrots is 1.25 mg/kg administered twice daily.[29] Experiences in diseased birds indicate that the use of enalapril in birds with cardiovascular disorders is of high therapeutic value. The authors treated cardiac insufficiencies and hydropericardium in birds with good results with extended administration of 5 mg/kg/d of longer than 1 year. Side effects were limited to an increase in packed cell volume (PCV) and signs of dehydration, which vanished with a dosage reduction to 1 mg/kg administered orally twice daily. For initial therapy of heart insufficiency in birds, a combination of glycosides, ACE blockers, and diuretics seems to be most beneficial.

Calcium sensitizers have been used in birds empirically (0.25 and 0.5 mg/kg/d), but to the authors' knowledge, their use has not been published. In birds with heart dilatation and pericardial effusion, the drug does not seem to have the same positive effect as is seen after treatment with ACE blockers.

Furosemide (0.1–0.2 mg/kg/d administered orally or intramuscularly) has a diuretic effect in birds, although the exact pharmacodynamic mechanism is still unknown. Indications are edema and pericardial effusion. Cardiac work is eased as a result of reduced pre- and afterload. Extended administration may lead to a potassium deficiency, which can cause heart arrhythmias. Treated birds should also be observed for dehydration. In the authors' experience, diuretics are primarily indicated for the initial therapy of cardiac insufficiency with fluid accumulation (eg, ascites, pericardial effusion) in combination with ACE blockers or glycosides.

Pericardiocentesis

Pericardiocentesis should be performed in birds with high-grade pericardial effusion. The removal of fluid from the pericardial cavity improves cardiac function. Guided by ultrasound, it is an easy and safe procedure that should be combined with diuretics and ACE blockers or glycosides.[30] Using ultrasonography to visualize the pericardial cavity, the needle is placed on the midline directly caudal to the sternum and pushed forward craniodorsally toward the heart. Removed fluid should not exceed 10 mL/kg of body mass per day to prevent hypovolemic shock. Puncture of the liver is necessary for this procedure but does not seem to have a negative effect. This procedure should only be done under isoflurane anesthesia to reduce the risk for sudden movements.

Adjunctive Therapy

Adjunctive therapy is essential to maintain organ function and circulatory activity. In addition to the heart, the function of the liver and kidneys may be affected because of circulatory insufficiencies. The liver may be congested, and renal blood flow may be reduced. The function of the lungs may also be affected as a primary cause for heart disease (fibrosis, and therefore increased pulmonary pressure) or secondary attributable to congestion. Cardiac therapy also affects these organs; for example, renal function is supported by the use of ACE blockers, and congestion of liver and lungs may be reduced through improved cardiac function (decreased preload). As supportive measures, birds should be incubated in a warm environment (approximately 25°C or higher), with sufficient air humidity (60% or greater). Stress should be reduced to a minimum. Fluid administration is essential when starting therapy. This is of importance to prevent circulatory collapse and shock, and, additionally, to prevent dehydration when using ACE blockers or diuretics. Substitution with electrolytes, vitamins, amino acids, and buffer solution may also be indicated. In case of suspected arteriosclerosis, support with vitamin A, vitamin C, vitamin E, and selenium is recommended.

SUMMARY

The avian heart is a high-performance organ that meets the enormous demands of being able to fly. Pathologic alterations are regularly found in pet birds in postmortem studies. Common findings include cardiomyopathy, pericardial effusion, and atherosclerosis. Physical examination parameters, such as auscultation and percussion, are minimally useful in the avian patient, but imaging techniques can give important information for diagnosis and therapy. In addition to radiography and ECG, the ultrasound examination is a useful technique for the assessment of cardiac function. Although therapeutic experiences are limited in comparison to mammals, recent studies show the value of ACE inhibitors and other drugs for the therapy of cardiovascular disease in birds.

REFERENCES

1. Orosz S. Anatomy of the cardiovascular system. In: Altman RB, Clubb SL, Dorrestein GM, Quesenberry K, editors. Avian medicine and surgery. Philadelphia: WB Saunders; 1997. p. 489–90.
2. Smith FM, West NH, Jones DR. The cardiovascular system. In: Whittow GC, editor. Sturkie's avian physiology. 5th edition. San Diego (CA): Academic Press; 2000. p. 141–232.
3. Orosz S. The avian cardiovascular system: anatomy and physiology for the clinician. Proceedings of the 25th Annual Association of Avian Veterinarians Conference, Avian Specialty Advanced Program. New Orleans (LA): Association of Avian Veterinarians; 2004. p. 3–10.
4. Oglesbee BL, Oglesbee MJ. Results of postmortem examination of psittacine birds with cardiac disease: 26 cases (1991–1995). J Am Vet Med Assoc 1998; 212(11):1737–42.
5. Krautwald-Junghanns ME, Braun S, Pees M, et al. Research on the anatomy and pathology of the psittacine heart. J Avian Med Surg 2004;18(1):2–11.
6. Krautwald-Junghanns ME, Pees M. Advances in diagnosing cardiac diseases. Proceedings of the 25th Annual Association of Avian Veterinarians Conference, Avian Specialty Advanced Program. New Orleans (LA): Association of Avian Veterinarians; 2004. p. 25–34.

7. Straub J, Pees M, Krautwald-Junghanns ME. Measurement of the cardiac silhouette in psittacines. J Am Vet Med Assoc 2002;221:76–9.

8. Hanley SH, Helen GM, Torrey S, et al. Establishing cardiac measurement standards in three avian species. J Avian Med Surg 1997;11:15–9.

9. Vink-Nooteboom M, Schoemaker NJ, Kik MJL, et al. Clinical diagnosis of aneurysm of the right coronary artery in a white cockatoo (Cacatua alba). J Small Anim Pract 1998;39:533–7.

10. Fischer I, Christen C, Scharf G, et al. Cardiomegaly in a whooper swan (Cygnus cygnus). Vet Rec 2005;156(6):178–82.

11. Pees M, Krautwald-Junghanns ME, Straub J. Evaluating and treating the cardiovascular system. In: Harrison GJ, Lightfoot T, editors. Avian veterinary compendium. Palm Beach (FL): Spix Publishing; 2006. p. 379–94.

12. Krautwald-Junghanns ME, Schulz M, Hagner D, et al. Transcoelomic two-dimensional echocardiography in the avian patient. J Avian Med Surg 1995;9: 19–31.

13. Pees M, Straub J, Krautwald-Junghanns ME. Echocardiographic examinations of 60 African grey parrots and 30 other psittacine birds. Vet Rec 2004;155(3):73–6.

14. Boskovic M, Krautwald-Junghanns ME, Failing K, et al. Möglichkeiten und Grenzen echokardiographischer Untersuchungen bei Tag- und Nachtgreifvögeln (Accipitriformes, Falconiformes, Strigiformes). Tierarztl Prax 1995;27:334–41.

15. Krautwald-Junghanns ME, Pees M, Schütterle N. Echokardiographische Untersuchungen an unsedierten Brieftauben (Columbia livia f. domestica) unter besonderer Berücksichtigung des Trainingszustandes. Berl Munch Tierarztl Wochenschr 2001;114:1–4.

16. Straub J, Forbes N, Pees M, et al. Pulsed-wave Doppler derived velocity of diastolic ventricular inflow and systolic aortic outflow in diurnal and nocturnal raptors. Vet Rec 2004;154(5):145–7.

17. Straub J, Forbes N, Pees M, et al. Effect of handling-induced stress on the results of spectral Doppler-echocardiography in falcons. Res Vet Sci 2003;74(2):119–22.

18. Pees M, Straub J, Schumacher J, et al. Pilotstudie zu echokardiographischen Untersuchungen mittels Farb- und pulsed-wave-Spektraldoppler an Blaukronenamazonen (Amazona ventralis) und Blaustirnamazonen (Amazona a. aestiva). Dtsch Tierarztl Wochenschr 2005;112(2):39–43.

19. Rosenthal K, Miller M. Cardiac disease. In: Altman RB, Clubb SL, Dorrestein GM, Quesenberry K, editors. Avian medicine and surgery. Philadelphia: WB Saunders; 1997. p. 491–500.

20. Aguilar RF, Smith VE, Ogburn P, et al. Arrhythmias associated with isoflurane anaesthesia in bald eagles (Haliaeetus leucocephalus). J Zoo Wildl Med 1995; 26(4):508–16.

21. Lumeij JT, Ritchie BW. Cardiovascular system. In: Ritchie BW, Harrison GJ, Harrison LR, editors. Avian medicine, principles and application. Lake Worth (FL): Wingers Publishing; 1994. p. 694–722.

22. Lumeij JT, Stokhof AA. Electrocardiogram of the racing pigeon (Columbia livia forma domestica). Res Vet Sci 1985;38:275–8.

23. Nap AM, Lumeij JT, Stokhof AA. Electrocardiogram of the African grey (Psittacus erithacus) and Amazon (Amazona sp.) parrot. Avian Pathol 1992;21:45–53.

24. Casares M, Enders F, Montaya JA. Electrocardiography in some macaw species (genus Anodorhynchus and Ara). Proceedings of the European Association of Avian Veterinarians Conference. Pisa (Italy): European Association of Avian Veterinarians; 1999. p. 158–63.

25. Hamlin RL, Stalnaker PS. Basis for use of digoxin in small birds. J Vet Pharmacol Ther 1987;10:354–6.
26. Wilson RC, Zenoble RD, Horton CR, et al. Single dose digoxin pharmacokinetics in Quaker conure. J Zoo Wildl Med 1989;20:432–4.
27. Pauletto P, Vescovo G, Scannapieco G, et al. Cardioprotection by beta blockers: molecular and structural aspects in experimental hypertension. Drugs Exp Clin Res 1990;16:123–8.
28. Pauletto P, Pessina AC, Pagnan A, et al. Evidence of reduced atherosclerotic lesions in broad breasted white turkeys treated with oxprenolol. Artery 1985;12: 220–33.
29. Pees M, Kuhring K, Demiraij F. et al. Bioavailability and compatibility of enalapril in birds. Proceedings of the 27th Annual Association of Avian Veterinarians Conference. San Antonio (TX): Association of Avian Veterinarians; 2006. p. 7–12.
30. Straub J, Pees M, Enders F, et al. Pericardiocentesis and the use of enalapril in a fisher's lovebird. Vet Rec 2003;152:24–6.

Cardiovascular Anatomy, Physiology, and Disease of Rodents and Small Exotic Mammals

J. Jill Heatley, DVM, MS, DABVP–Avian, DACZM

KEYWORDS
- Cardiovascular • Rodent • Marsupial • Hedgehog
- Skunk • Disease

Cardiovascular disease in the small exotic mammals is anecdotally common, but clinical reports of diagnosis and treatment of disease are rare. This article focuses on known causes of cardiovascular disease in the small exotic mammal. Normal anatomy and physiology, as it differs from the dog and cat, is also highlighted. Cardiomyopathy, dirofilariasis, atrial thrombosis, and other acquired and congenital cardiac and vascular diseases of rodents, hedgehogs, sugar gliders, raccoons, opossums, and skunks are reviewed. Neoplastic diseases are not included. Expected clinical signs and diagnostic and treatment options, including a formulary, are provided for these species. This article is intended to stimulate the exotic mammal practitioner to diagnose, treat, and report cases of cardiovascular disease in these species. Little information in this article is new; however, the reader may find valuable resources because some of these species were anatomically and physiologically studied in the 1970s. This review also points out the dearth of baseline information available for some of these species.

CARDIOVASCULAR ANATOMY AND PHYSIOLOGY

This section reviews normal clinically applied cardiovascular and anatomy and physiology of small exotic mammals. Most information is limited to the heart and great vessels of the common rodents, the North American opossum (*Monodelphis virginianus*), the sugar glider (*Petaurus breviceps*), raccoon (*Procyonis lotor*), and the skunk (*Mephitis* and *Spilogale* spp). Much information is available for laboratory rodents but information on the cardiovascular anatomy and physiology of wildlife species is limited. Ranges for respiratory and heart rates are given in **Table 1**.

Department of Small Animal Clinical Sciences, Zoological Medicine Service, College of Veterinary Medicine, Texas A&M University, College Station, TX 77843-4474, USA
E-mail address: jheatley@cvm.tamu.edu

Vet Clin Exot Anim 12 (2009) 99–113
doi:10.1016/j.cvex.2008.08.006
1094-9194/08/$ – see front matter © 2009 Elsevier Inc. All rights reserved.

vetexotic.theclinics.com

Table 1
Normal respiratory and heart rates for small exotic mammals

Species	Respiratory Rate (Breaths/Min)	Heart Rate (Beats/Min)
Mouse	60–220	310–840
Rat	115	250–500
Hamster	35–135	250–500
Gerbil	90	360
Guinea pig	40–100	230–380
Chinchilla	20–80	137–201
Prairie dog	40–60	83–318
Hedgehog	20–50	180–260
Sugar glider	16–40	180–300
Opossum	—	180–300
Skunk	—	140–190
Raccoon	—	94–134

Data from Refs. [2,3,18,23,31,54,68,69]

In the mouse (*Mus musculus*), the heart extends from ribs three to six in its ventral-most aspects.[1] Healthy mouse systolic blood pressures range from 84 to 105 mm Hg and are not affected by increases in body temperature. Heart rate and cardiac output change based on the animal's body size, however. There are also wide variations in heart rate and blood pressure based on the strain of mouse.[2]

The heart of the rat (*Rattus norvegicus*) is located on the midline in the thorax, apex near the diaphragm, with the lateral aspects bounded by the lungs.[1] The small left lung size of the rat exposes the heart to the left thoracic wall between the third and fifth ribs and facilitates visualization of the heart for venipuncture. Rats have two cranial vena cavae: the right cranial vena cava empties the right atrium and the left cranial vena cava is joined by the azygos vein and the caudal vena cava and then enters the right atrium. Of the rodents, rats have the thinnest pulmonary artery and the thickest pulmonary vein. Cardiac striated muscle in the rat extends to lung tissue, which makes these species particularly susceptible to infectious agents spread between the heart, pulmonary veins, and lungs. Blood supply to the heart of the rat differs from other mammals and is largely extracoronary from branches of the internal mammary and subclavian arteries.[3] Normal cardiovascular parameters of the rat include a systolic blood pressure of 116 mm Hg and a diastolic blood pressure of 90 mm Hg.

In the hamster (*Mesocricetus auratus*), the heart is found on the midline, contacts the thoracic wall from ribs three to five, and is not obscured ventrally by a lung lobe on the right or left.[1] The aortic arch has three branches: the innominate, the left common carotid, and the left subclavian. This species also has three caval veins: two cranial vena cavae and one caudal vena cava. Like some other rodent species, the hamster also has sheaths of cardiac fibers in its pulmonary vessel walls. The hamster has cartilaginous foci in the central fibrous body of the heart that act as pivots to resist mechanical tensions of the cardiac cycle. Normal deposition of calcium in the extracellular matrix of these foci reinforces the cartilaginous tissue and is not an age-related change.[4]

Gerbil (*Meriones unguiculatus*) cardiovascular anatomy is considered similar to other rodents except that many gerbils lack a complete Circle of Willis, an anastomosis of arteries at the base of brain. This vascular anatomy makes gerbils susceptible to cerebral ischemia on ligation of the common carotid artery and valuable as models for stroke research (forebrain ischemia). Recent evidence indicates that this cerebrovascular anatomy varies based on the gerbil supplier, however, and up to 40% of gerbils may have some brain base arterial anastomosis.[5]

Guinea pigs (*Cavia porcellus*) are noted for their spectacular collateralization of their coronary arteries, making them unlikely to develop myocardial infarction. Guinea pigs have lower basal and peak coronary blood flow than the rat, however. Guinea pigs are a preferred species for the studies of human cardiac disease based on their docile nature and ease of obtaining ECG recordings, which mimic that of humans.[6] The guinea pig heart sound normally consists of the standard two sounds of lub (louder)/dub (softer) but may be normally preceded by a fourth heart sound corresponding to atrial contraction.[7] The guinea pig heart normally lies on the midline and extends from the second to the fourth intercostal space.[8] The lumen of the right ventricle of the guinea pig contains a moderator band. The guinea pig heart occupies a relatively large space in the thorax and is therefore surrounded by relatively small lung space. There are two pericardial layers; the outer is more fibrous, whereas the inner is a thinner serous layer. For venipuncture in this species and the chinchilla, the cranial vena cava is not recommended based on proximity of the heart and major vessels in the relatively compact thorax and the attendant risk for laceration of these structures.

Anatomic studies of the cardiac anatomy of the chinchilla (*Chinchilla laniger*) are limited. Based on anatomic preparation and gross dissection of chinchillas, the left coronary artery is the sole artery to supply the heart with blood. The right coronary artery is absent in chinchillas.[9] The cardiac ganglia of the chinchilla are localized on the epicardium of the ventral surface of the right atria.[10]

The cardiovascular anatomy of the woodchuck (*Marmota monax*) has been extensively studied based on their use as laboratory animals.[11] This species has a cone-shaped heart with a broad base and a narrow apex. The heart is obliquely aligned in the thorax with its longitudinal axis 45 degrees from center and the apex caudally displaced to the left. In a 2.7-kg woodchuck, the heart measures 35 mm in length, 25 mm in width, and weighs 7 g. The heart extends within the thorax from the second intercostal space to the cranial border of the fifth rib. The pulmonary and aortic valves consist of three semilunar valvules and the right atrioventricular valve consists of three leaflets or cusps. Woodchucks have two cranial caval veins.

The prairie dog (*Cyonomys ludivicianus*) is considered a primitive sciurid with a unilobate left lung.[12] The heart lies in the midline of the body with the apex directed toward the left. Information about the cardiovascular system and physiology of the hedgehog is limited to *Erinaceus europeus*.[13] In this species, there is a limitation of the sinoatrial node to the right of the sinoatrial junction; thus the sinoatrial node and atrioventricular node are not connected. The heart valves are mainly muscular and the interatrial septum is characterized as a very thin layer of fibrous tissue. There is cartilage in the heart base. Although some insectivore species have been found to possess cardiac-like muscle in the intrapulmonary vein (similar to the rat), this has not been investigated in any hedgehog species.[14]

Marsupials included here are the sugar glider (*P breviceps*) and the North American opossum (*D virginiana*). Several features of the marsupial heart are considered primitive and closer in form to birds, reptiles, and monotremes than to other mammals. The right ventricle is crescent shaped in transverse section and wraps around the left ventricle.[15] There is only a single leaflet of the atrioventricular valve.[15] The cardiac veins and arteries also pursue a course more similar to that of birds than placental mammals. The right atrium is generally bifurcated with one appendage of the auricle in front and one behind the ascending aorta; however, the functional significant of this bifurcation remains uninvestigated. In general marsupials have a slower metabolism than eutherian mammals by about two thirds; this results in about half the rate of heart beats per minute and for compensatory blood volume a 30% heavier marsupial heart. The expected marsupial heart rate can be estimated based on animal size. A 20- to 40-g animal would be expected to have 449 to 378 beats per minute (bpm), a 100- to 250-g animal (most adult sugar gliders fit into this range) 239 to 300 bpm, a 400-g to 1-kg animal 212 to 169 bpm, a 1.5- to 2-kg animal 142 to 151 bpm, and a 3- to 5-kg marsupial would have an expected heart rate of 113 to 128 bpm.[16]

CARDIOVASCULAR DISEASES OF THE RODENT

Common cardiovascular diseases vary based on the species and strain. Based on literature review and clinical practice, gerbils, hamsters, guinea pigs, chinchillas, and prairie dogs can develop cardiovascular disease. Rats and mice seem overall less prone to cardiac disease.

Causes of cardiac disease in mice include dystrophic mineralization, atrial thrombosis, amyloidosis, vitamin deficiency, septicemia, and rancid feed. Naturally occurring mineralization of the myocardium and epicardium of the left ventricle and interventricular system is a common finding at necropsy in some inbred strains of mice. Mineralization may be accompanied by fibrosis and mononuclear inflammatory infiltrates. Mild lesions may be incidental findings at necropsy but severe lesions may affect myocardial function. Deficiencies in vitamin E or choline may also cause heart failure or myocardial lesions. Cardiomyopathy has a high incidence in certain mouse strains, suggesting a genetic component. These mice may have dystrophic cardiac calcification and may be more prone to the development of septicemia. A laboratory colony of mice inadvertently fed rancid feed suffered diarrhea and death and at necropsy were found to have myocarditis. Atrial thrombosis is strain-related and more common in aged mice. Atrial thrombosis usually occurs in the left atrium and auricle and may be accompanied by amyloidosis. Amyloid is also commonly deposited in the great vessels. Clinical signs of cardiac disease in mice include severe dyspnea, tachypnea, and abdominal distension. Periarteritis occurs in aged mice.[2]

Causes of cardiac disease in the rat include cardiomyopathy, atrial thrombosis, aortic mineralization secondary to nephropathy, coronary arteriosclerosis, endocardial hyperplasia, endocardiosis, and toxicity. Coronary arteriosclerosis is relatively uncommon in the rat. Chronic myocardial disease is a major cause of death in aged male rats of multiple strains when fed ad libitum. This disease, also known as cardiomyopathy or chronic progressive cardiomyopathy, may be observed as early as 3 months of age. Both dilated and hypertrophic forms of cardiomyopathy occur. In the dilated form, the heart may be grossly enlarged with pale streaks in the myocardium. Increased heart weight correlates with degree of histologic damage. Necrosis of myocardial fibers and interstitial infiltration of mononuclear cells occurs with fibrosis, a more prominent late-stage finding. The incidence of cardiomyopathy in the rat is reduced by moderate (25% to 30%) dietary restriction.[3] Myocardial mineralization and aortic mineralization are often found in rats secondary to nephropathy. Endocardial hyperplasia commonly occurs in the aged rat when thickening and proliferation of the subendocardium due to sarcoma, schwannoma, or fibroelastosis expands into the ventricular lumen. Endocardiosis or myxomatous thickening of the heart valves may also result in congestive heart failure in the rat. Clinical signs of congestive heart failure in the rat include edema, ascites, cardiomegaly, and lethargy. Cardiodegeneration was caused by administration of *Senna occidentalis* seeds to rats that became lethargic, weak, recumbent, depressed, and emaciated.[17]

Cardiovascular diseases of the gerbil include ventricular septal heart defect, hyperadrenocorticism cardiovascular disease complex, focal myocardial degeneration, myocarditis/endocarditis, atrial thrombosis, and pulmonary microthrombi. Although gerbils tend toward lipemia even while on a low-fat diet, high cholesterol of gerbils has not been associated with atherosclerosis. In newborn gerbils ventricular septal defect has been reported.[18] A hyperadrenocorticism/cardiovascular disease complex affects only breeding gerbils. At necropsy aortic plaques and mineralization of the aortic, mesenteric, renal, and peripheral arteries occur. Additionally, enlarged pancreatic islets, hepatic lipidosis, thymic involution, and adrenal lipid depletions are also noted. Affected animals may have diabetes, obesity, elevated triglycerides, and occasionally functional pheochromocytomas. Focal myocardial degeneration is reported most commonly in breeding gerbils. Affected hearts at necropsy have focal myocardial necrosis fibrosis and ischemic lesions.

A recent pathology review of pet Syrian hamsters (*Mesocricetus auratus*) indicated a 6% incidence of cardiac disease, although this may be an underestimate based on lack of submission of the heart in many cases.[19] Noninfectious diseases of pet and laboratory hamsters include various congenital abnormalities, cardiomyopathy, atrial thrombosis, calcifying vasculopathy, and myocardial mineralization. Tyzzer disease (*Bacillus piliformis*) and *Salmonella enteritidis* can also cause cardiovascular disease in the hamster. Hamster incidence of atrial thrombosis is up to 73% in some laboratory strains. Pathophysiology is believed to progress from cardiomyopathy to left atrial thrombosis to eventual death from consumptive coagulopathy. Clinical signs of atrial thrombosis are generally referable to those caused by cardiomyopathy and include hyperpnea, tachycardia, and cyanosis. Androgens protect from heart disease in the hamster; thus female hamsters tend to suffer cardiovascular disease earlier ($\sim$13.5 months) than males ($\sim$21.5 months). Neutering male hamsters removes this effect. Cardiomyopathy is more common in the aged (>1.5 years) hamster. In the laboratory setting, both dilated and cardiomyopathic types of cardiomyopathy occur in certain hamster strains and are related to defects in the same gene.[20,21] Clinical signs of cardiovascular disease in the hamster may be nonspecific but include cold extremities, lethargy, anorexia, and tachypnea. In other hamster species, less information is available; the Chinese hamster (*Cricetulus griseus*), may suffer arteriosclerosis, myocarditis, myocardial fibrosis, and auricular thrombosis.[19] When clinical signs occur, hamsters with cardiovascular disease may be expected to live only about 7 days without treatment.

Cardiovascular diseases reported in the guinea pig include cardiomyopathy, rhabdomyomatosis, pericardial effusion, toxicity, and metastatic or dystrophic mineralization.[22] Dyspnea, tachypnea, tachycardia, pale mucous membranes, and acute onset of weakness have been reported as clinical signs of cardiac dysfunction in the guinea pig.[22] Dystrophic mineralization causes mineralization of cardiac muscle of cardiac fibers and muscles throughout the body in guinea pigs and may be asymptomatic in guinea pigs older than 1 year of age. Irregular gray patches of mineral composed of calcium phosphate or carbonate and other minerals maybe deposited in many organs and muscles, including the aorta. Causes of this inappropriate mineral deposition may include low local tissue pH, magnesium deficiency, or diets high in calcium and phosphate and low in magnesium. Clinical signs include poor growth, muscle stiffness, bone deformities, nephrosis, and death. Rhabdomyomatosis is also common in guinea pigs but causes no apparent cardiac impairment and is caused by a congenital defect of metabolism. Glycogen accumulation in myofibers of the heart appears as pale pink foci or streaks commonly found in the left ventricle. *Nerium oleander* ingestion can cause cardiac dysrhythmias in the guinea pig, among other signs, and may be treated successfully with appropriate supportive care.[23]

Prairie dogs 3 to 4 years of age may develop dilated cardiomyopathy.[24] Clinical signs include dyspnea, lethargy, and anorexia. Odontoma, pneumonia, and obesity must be assessed as rule-outs or complicating factors. Treatment may be unrewarding; a nutritional cause is proposed. A lipoma that encompassed the carotid arteries, jugular veins, and thymus was found in the cranial mediastinum of a 3-year-old prairie dog. Clinical signs included dysphagia, weight loss, dyspnea, and eventually death.[18]

Chinchilla cardiovascular disease may be common, based on practitioner anecdotal reports.[25] Apparently normal chinchillas have cardiac murmurs during routine physical examination. Cardiomyopathy has been reported in two young black velvet female chinchillas. Ventricular septal defect and tricuspid regurgitation have also been reported in a single male 2-year-old chinchilla.[26] This animal lacked apparent clinical signs at diagnosis but died at approximately 16 months of age. Necropsy findings included papillary muscle dysplasia and mitral valve malformation. Acute death of a related chinchilla may also have been attributable to cardiac disease. Appropriate diagnostics are warranted in any chinchilla with cardiac abnormalities.

Diseases affecting the cardiovascular system are common in woodchucks and include white muscle disease, capture myopathy, nutritional deficiency, cardiomyopathy, vegetative endocarditis, arteriosclerosis, aortic rupture, cerebrovascular hemorrhage, and cardiac tamponade.[27] Parasites may also affect the cardiovascular system in woodchucks, including *Sarcocystis* spp, *Baylisascaris* spp, and *Taenia mustelae*.[28] White muscle disease may affect the heart of newly captured woodchucks as part of capture myopathy complex or based on nutritional deficiency of woodchucks in captivity several weeks. Clinical signs stem from generalized muscle disease and include weakness, lethargy, and reluctance to move. Histologic lesions range from muscle swelling and breakage to mineralization and muscle atrophy and fibrosis in chronic cases. Mild manifestations may respond to supplementation with vitamin E and supportive care, and death may occur in severe cases. Aortic rupture occurs in wild-caught and laboratory-reared woodchucks. There are no premonitory signs and no gender predisposition, although death from aortic rupture occurs in older woodchucks. Systemic hypertension may be a contributory factor, because concurrent glomerulonephritis or interstitial nephritis is often found in these cases. Cardiomyopathy resulting in congestive heart failure may be the most common disease of woodchucks. Clinical signs include respiratory distress, ascites, subcutaneous edema, muffled heart sounds, heart murmurs, and heart arrhythmias. Animals may also suffer sudden death without premonitory signs. At necropsy these animals often have a grossly enlarged heart ($32.3 \text{ g} \pm 5.4 \text{ g}$) compared with other woodchucks ($11.6 \text{ g} \pm 2.8 \text{ g}$).[27]

CARDIOVASCULAR DISEASES OF THE HEDGEHOG AND SUGAR GLIDER

Incidence of cardiovascular disease in the African hedgehog (*Atelerix albiventris*) approaches 40%.[29] Geriatric males are more likely to have cardiac disease but reports of affected animals include those as young as 1 year of age. Acute death may occur but many animals exhibit clinical signs, such as heart murmur, moist rales, dyspnea, dehydration, weight loss, and lethargy. Cardiomegaly, hepatomegaly, pulmonary edema, or congestion, hydrothorax, ascites, and pulmonary or renal infarcts are common gross necropsy findings.[29,30] Possible causes of cardiac disease in the hedgehog include diet, toxin, stress, obesity, and genetics. Cardiac disease and myonecrosis have been reported in sugar gliders in association with malnutrition.[31]

CARDIOVASCULAR DISEASES OF THE SKUNK, OPOSSUM, AND RACCOON

Most reports of cardiovascular disease in the skunk (*M mephitis*), opossum (*D virginiana*), and raccoon (*P lotor*) are limited to experimental models, wildlife necropsies, and anecdotal mention. Cardiomyopathies are considered a serious health concern of animals older than 2 years of age when kept in captivity, likely based on resultant obesity.[32–34] Dilated and hypertrophic forms of cardiomyopathy occur in these species.[31] No current clinical report of treatment of cardiovascular disease in these species was found by the author. In the experimental setting, the opossum is a model for endocarditis and naturally occurring endocarditis and septicemia have also been reported.[35–40] The layman's term "crispy ear" is given to a disease, also called dermal septic necrosis, affecting the ears and tail tips of affected opossums that have clinical signs of septicemia and necrosis of the affected areas. The cause of this apparently vascular disease has not been scientifically investigated. Streptococcal endocarditis and associated vasculitis should be considered in young heterothermic animals with these clinical signs. The opossum has also been used as a scientific model for investigation of systemic hypertension.[41]

Trypanosoma cruzi infection occurs in skunks, raccoons, and oppossums.[37,42–44] In experimental infection of the skunk, animals showed minimal clinical signs but evidenced chronic granulomatous myocarditis.[42] Raccoons infected with this organism in Georgia seem to suffer little cardiovascular pathology.[43] Infection prevalence of trypanosomiasis among North American wildlife is highest among raccoons (16%) and opossums (38%).[45] A single case of cor pulmonale and cardiac failure has been reported in an adult male captive spotted skunk (*Spilogale putorius*), which died. No treatment or diagnostics specific to cardiovascular disease were performed in this skunk, which evidenced signs of dyspnea, anorexia, lethargy, and dried nasal exudates and had a history of tooth abscessation.[46] *Streptococcus equisimilis* and *Streptococcus canis* were isolated from purulent myocarditis in a wild radio-collared skunk that was found dead.[47]

Immature *Dirofilaria immitis* were found naturally occurring in one raccoon.[48] Experimental inoculation of raccoons suggests, and additional data from wild raccoon supports, the hypothesis that raccoons are not particularly susceptible to *Dirofilaria immitis* infection.[48–51] The susceptibility of skunks and opossums to Dirofilariasis has not been definitively established but they are believed to be susceptible.[33]

DIAGNOSIS OF CARDIOVASCULAR DISEASE IN THE SMALL EXOTIC MAMMAL

Assessment of the cardiovascular system can be challenging, especially in the more diminutive species. A careful observational examination along with administration of blow-by oxygen can be rewarding. Observation of the cardiac impulse by auscultation and by placement of the finger on the chest or by assessment with Doppler probe to make cardiac sounds more audible is recommended. Perfusion may be assessed by observation of the feet, tail, and ears for color and temperature. Make careful note of baseline heart rate and respiratory rate of the patient to later facilitate the patient response to therapy. ECG reference ranges have been obtained in mice and other small quadrupeds noninvasively by placement of the feet on platform-embedded electrodes.[52] Diagnostics for use in cardiovascular disease of the small exotic mammal can be adapted from the companion mammal with knowledge of normal physiology of the species at hand.

ECG

Normal ECG tracing values have been reported for the guinea pig, raccoon, and opossum (**Table 2**).[7,53–57] Guinea pig electrocardiogram tracings are valued because they

Table 2
Reference values for ECG parameters in small exotic mammals

Parameter (Units)	Guinea Pig[7]	Raccoon[a,53]	Opossum[59]
P wave duration (sec)	0.015–0.035	—	0.025–0.035
P wave amplitude (mV)	0.01	0.003–0.023	0.005–0.011[a]
P-R interval (sec)	0.048–0.060	—	0.06–0.08
QRS duration (sec)	0.008–0.046	0.037–0.050	0.030–0.060
R wave amplitude (mV)	1.1–1.9	0.042–0.390	0.040–0.080[a]
QT interval (sec)	0.106–0.144	0.220±0.178	0.14–0.018
T wave amplitude (mV)	0.062	0.011–0.149	0.010–0.020[a]
Mean electrical axis (degrees)	+20 to +80	—	—

Most animals anesthetized and in right lateral recumbency, Lead II.
 [a] Range adapted from lead AvF.
Data from Refs.[7,53,59]

closely resemble the human compared with other lab rodents. The guinea pig's attitude provides unrestrained electrode measurements; this animal will freely stand on a plate electrode to obtain tracings.[7]

The opossum ECG has been studied based on its use as a research model. Heart rate and ECG wave configurations, intervals, and amplitudes are not affected by death feigning in the opossum.[58] ECG tracing measurements from 10 apparently healthy wild-caught opossums that were anesthetized in right lateral recumbence are given (see **Table 2**).[53] Gender and position did not affect ECG recordings in this species. Sinus respiratory arrhythmia was present in the lightly anesthetized or unanesthetized opossums. The P wave of the opossum may be positive or negative in Lead II. Anesthetized raccoons have similar QRS vector orientation to that of the dog but low QRS amplitude similar to cats.[59] New technology is available for noninvasive measurement of ECG in conscious mice based on very small electrodes embedded in a platform on which the patient stands. This system includes software for analysis, and although not yet available for clinical use the system has already determined gender and age differences in mouse heart rates.[52]

Radiographs

Anatomic and radiographic atlases are available for normal reference for rodents and other small mammals.[60,61] In the guinea pig the heart is rather cranially placed and has a ventrocranial inclination; this species also normally has a rather wide mediastinum.[61] Cardiogenic edema may be evident by increased pulmonary density and tracheal elevation due to cardiac enlargement may occur.[61] On radiographic images of the normal Syrian hamster, the apex of the heart points caudoventrally and to the left.[61]

In the hedgehog, normal radiographic cardiac size or ultrasonographic parameters have not yet been reported. Common radiographic findings associated with cardiac disease in these species generally mimic those of small companion animals, however: pleural edema, pleural effusion, aerophagia, and tracheal elevation occurs. In the mouse and rat, the heart silhouette can only be distinguished caudally from the lung lobes based on the cranial, persistent thymus.[60] The rat has a relatively wide cranial mediastinum also.

Ultrasound

In the small exotic mammal, ultrasound may be most useful to determine the type of cardiac dysfunction and the presence of a mass, dirofilariasis, or lung consolidation.

Ultrasonographic parameters of normal subjects have been determined for the mouse, Syrian hamster, rabbit, guinea pig, ferret, and chinchilla (**Table 3**). In chinchilla and mouse anesthesia, and anesthetic type affects ultrasonographic parameters.[25,62-64] On ultrasonography, a fractional shortening of less than 25% has been reported as consistent with cardiac dysfunction in the hedgehog.[65] Normal ultrasonographic parameters have not been determined for the skunk, raccoon, opossum, prairie dog, gray squirrel, or sugar glider.

Other Diagnostics

Appropriate serology for infectious disease that may affect these species, such as pasteurellosis, trypanosomiasis, and dirofilariasis, may be used. In the author's hands, serologic detection of heartworms in ferrets by an antigen test has been a successful antemortem diagnostic based on necropsy and ultrasonographic findings. Thoracocentesis or pleurocentesis is diagnostically useful, especially in ruling out infectious and neoplastic causes of effusion. MRI has been used to assess cardiomyopathic disease of hamsters.

TREATMENT OF CARDIOVASCULAR DISEASE IN THE SMALL EXOTIC MAMMAL

Treatment of cardiovascular disease in small exotic mammals is largely extrapolated from data obtained from the cat, dog, and ferret.[31] Valuable information may also be obtained from the laboratory animal literature, wherein rodent species are used for cardiovascular research. For example, verapamil may be the drug of choice for cardiomyopathic hamsters based on comparison of propranolol and digoxin, because only verapamil preserves cardiac contractility.[66] Additionally, chronic administration of enalapril and amlodipine prevent cardiac remodeling and reduce cardiac dysfunction in cardiomyopathic hamsters.[67] Recommended dosages for cardiac and vascular drugs in small exotic mammals, some extrapolated from experimental literature, are summarized in **Table 4**.

Table 3
Reference ultrasonographic measurements of small exotic mammals

Parameter (mm)	Mouse[70]	Hamster[71]	Rat[72]	Guinea Pig[73]	Chinchilla[25]
LVIDd	3.48–3.66	3.7–4.5	5.93–6.43	6.49–7.21	5.1–6.9
LVIDs	2.26–2.42	1.9–2.7	4.08–4.42	4.18–4.52	2.3–4.3
LVPWd	0.41–0.43	0.9–1.1	1.12–1.70	1.44–2.06	2.0–2.8
LVPWs	0.86–0.92		2.02–2.70	1.91–2.61	—
IVSd	0.42–0.44	0.9–1.1	1.06–1.36	1.88–2.68	1.5–2.3
IVSs	0.89–0.93		1.40–1.90	2.22–3.38	—
LA	—	—	—	4.61–5.29	4.3–5.9
AO	—	—	—	4.40–4.90	3.7–6.0

Range derived from mean ±1 SD, animals anesthetized in most instances.
Abbreviations: AO, aorta; d, diastolic; HR, heart rate; IVS, internal ventricular septum; LA, left atrium; LVID, left ventricular internal diameter; LVPW, left ventricular posterior wall; s, systolic.
Data from Refs.[25,70-73]

Table 4
Therapeutics for use in small exotic mammals with cardiovascular disease

Species	Drug	Dosage	Comments, indication
Hamster	Amlodipine	10 mg/kg/d in food	Calcium antagonist. Amlodipine prevents cell death and fibrosis and reduces cardiac dysfunction in cardiomyopathic hamsters.[67]
Rat	Atenolol	5 mg/kg[77]	β-blocker, hypertrophic cardiomyopathy. Prolongs filling, decreases myocardial ischemia.
Hamster, prairie dog	Digoxin	0.05–0.01 mg/kg PO q 12–24 h	Positive inotrope. Right-sided heart failure, nonresponsive cardiomyopathy, dilated cardiomyopathy. Also indicated for atrial fibrillation.
Hamster	Diltiazem	25 mg/kg/d orally[78]	Calcium channel blocker. Benzodiazepine like calcium antagonist. Increases ventricular filling, reduces heart rate and blood pressure, reduces myocardial oxygen consumption.
Hedgehog Hamster	Enalapril	0.5 mg/kg PO q 24—48 h 20 mg/kg/day in food[67]	Angiotensin-converting enzyme inhibitor. Balanced vasodilator; avoid use in animal with concurrent renal disease.
Chinchilla, guinea pig, hamster, mouse, rat Hedgehog Prairie dog	Furosemide	1–10 mg/kg IM, SQ, PO q 4–12 h 2.5–5.0 mg/kg q 8 h 1–4 mg/kg PO, SQ, q 12 h	Diuretic, reduction of ascites, pleural effusion, pulmonary edema.

Rodents	Isoprenaline	0.1–1 mg/kg/min IV, IC	Complete heart block, low cardiac output.
All	Nitroglycerin ointment 2%	1/16 in/kg. Apply to hairless region q 12–24 h. Total dose 5–10 μg/kg[77]	Initial adjunctive venodilation for emergency use
Rodents	Propranolol	0.1 mg/kg IV, IC	β-blocker, hypertrophic cardiomyopathy. Prolongs filling, decreases myocardial ischemia. Tachyarrhythmia
Rat	Pimobendan	1 mg/kg[79]	Phosphodiesterase inhibitor
All	Omega 3 oils in flax oil Coenzyme Q10 L-carnitine Taurine	25 mg/d 10–30 mg/d 25 mg/d 50 mg/d	Generally recommended nutraceuticals for cardiac support in rodents and small exotic mammals
Hamster Rat	Verapamil	0.25–0.5 mg/hamster SQ 5 mg/kg/d IP[80] 0.75 mg/mL in drinking water	Calcium channel blocker. Increases ventricular filling, reduces heart rate and blood pressure, reduces myocardial oxygen consumption.

Data from Refs. [69,74–76]

REFERENCES

1. Popesko P, Rajtova V, Horak J. A colour atlas of anatomy of small laboratory animals: rat, mouse, hamster. Bratislava: Elsevier; 1992.
2. Jacoby RO, Fox JG, Davisson M. Biology and diseases of mice. Laboratory Animal Medicine. 2nd edition. Boston: Academic Press; 2002. p. 35–120.
3. Kohn DF, Clifford CB. Biology and diseases of rats. In: Fox J, Anderson LC, Loew FM, et al, editors. Laboratory animal medicine. 2nd edition. Boston: Academic Press; 2002. p. 121–65.
4. Durán AC, López D, Guerrero A, et al. Formation of cartilaginous foci in the central fibrous body of the heart in Syrian hamsters (Mesocricetus auratus). J Anat 2004; 205:219–27.
5. Laidley DT, Colbourne F, Corbett D. Increased behavioural and histological variability arising from changes in cerebrovascular anatomy of the mongolian gerbil. Curr Neurovas Res 2005;2:401–7.
6. Hamlin RL. The guinea pig in cardiac safety pharmacology. J Pharmacol Toxicol Methods 2007;55:1–2.
7. Sisk DB. Physiology. In: Wagner JE, Manning PJ, editors. The biology of the guinea pig. San Diego: Academic Press; 1976. p. 63–92.
8. Cooper G, Schiller A. Anatomy of the guinea pig. Cambridge: Harvard Univeristy Press; 1975.
9. Ozdemir V, Cevik-Demirkan A, Turkmenoglu I. The right coronary artery is absent in the chinchilla (Chinchilla lanigera). Anat Histol Embryol 2008;37:114–7.
10. Kuder T, Nowak E, Szczurkowski A, et al. A comparative study on cardiac ganglia in midday gerbil, Egyptian spiny mouse, chinchilla laniger and pigeon. Anat Histol Embryol 2003;32:134–40.
11. Beziudenhout A, Evans H. Anatomy of the woodchuck (Marmota monax). Lawrence: Allen Press; 2005.
12. Dearden LC. The gross anatomy of the viscera of the prairie dog. J Mammal 1953;34:15–27.
13. Walls E. Specialized conducting tissue in the heart of the common hedgehog. (Erinaceus europaeus). J Anat 1943;77:294–8.
14. Endo H, MIfune H, Meada S, et al. Cardiac-like musculature of the intrapulmonary venous wall of the long-clawed shrew (Sorex unguiculatus), common tree shrew (Tipaia glis) and common marmoset (Callithrix jacchus). The Anatomical Record 1997;247:45–52.
15. Wade O, Neely P. The heart and attached vessels of the opossum, a marsupial. J Mammol 1949;30:111–6.
16. Johnson Delaney C. Marsupials. In: Johnson Delaney C, editor. Exotic companion medicine handbook for veterinarians. Lake Worth: Zoological Education Network; 2000.
17. Barbosa-Ferreira M, Dagli MLZ, Maiorka PC, et al. Sub-acute intoxication by Senna occidentalis seeds in rats. Food Chem Toxicol 2005;43:497–503.
18. Donnelly T, Quimby FW. Biology and diseases of other rodents. In: Fox J, Anderson LC, Loew FM, et al, editors. Laboratory animal medicine. 2nd edition. Boston: Academic Press; 2002. p. 248–91.
19. Schmidt RE, Reavill DR. Cardiovascular disease in hamsters: review and retrospective study. Journal of Exotic Pet Medicine 2007;16:49–51.
20. Sakamoto A. Electrical and ionic abnormalities in the heart of cardiomyopathic hamsters: in quest of a new paradigm for cardiac failure and lethal arrhythmia. Mol Cell Biochem 2004;259:183–7.

21. Sakamoto A, Ono K, Abe M, et al. Both hypertrophic and dilated cardiomyopathies are caused by mutation of the same gene, delta-sarcoglycan, in hamster: an animal model of disrupted dystrophin-associated glycoprotein complex. Proc Natl Acad Sci U S A 1997;94:13873–8.

22. Dyzban LA, Garrod LA, Besso J. Pericardial effusion and pericardiocentesis in a guinea pig (Cavia porcellus). J Am Anim Hosp Assoc 2001;37:21–6.

23. Harkness JE, Murray KA, Wagner JE, et al. Biology and diseases of guinea pigs. In: Fox J, Anderson LC, Loew FM, et al, editors. Laboratory animal medicine. Boston: Academic Press; 2002. p. 204–46.

24. Funk R. Medical management of prairie dogs. In: Quesenberry KE, Carpenter JW, editors. Ferrets, rabbits & rodents: clinical medicine and surgery. St. Louis (MO): Saunders; 2004. p. 266–73.

25. Linde A, Summerfield NJ, Johnston M, et al. Echocardiography in the chinchilla. J Vet Intern Med 2004;18:772–4.

26. Donnelly T. Disease problems of chinchillas. Philadelphia. In: Quesenberry KE, Carpenter JW, editors. Ferrets, rabbits & rodents: clinical medicine and surgery. St. Louis (MO): Saunders; 2004. p. 255–65.

27. Bellezza CA, Concannon PW, Hornbucke WE, et al. Woochucks as laboratory animals. In: Fox JG, Anderson LC, Loew FM, et al, editors. Laboratory animal medicine. 2nd edition. Boston: Academic Press; 2002. p. 309–27.

28. Roth L, King JM. Congestive cardiomyopathy in the woodchuck Marmota mona. J Wildl Dis 1986;22:533–7.

29. Raymond J, Garner M. Cardiomyopathy in captive African hedgehogs. J Vet Diagn Invest 2000;12:468–72.

30. Beurgelt CD. Histopathologic findings in pet hedgehogs with nonneoplastic conditions. Veterinary Medicine 2002;660–5.

31. Delayney CJ. Practical marsupial medicine. Association of Avian Veterinarians and Association of Exotic Mammal Veterinarians 2006;51–60.

32. Kramer MH, Lennox A. Exotic pet care: what veterinarians need to know about skunks. Exotic DVM 2003;5:36–41.

33. Fernandez-Moran J. Mustelidae. In: Fowler M, Miller R, editors. Zoo & wild animal medicine. Elsevier: St Louis; 2003. p. 501–17.

34. Johnson-Delaney C. Practical marsupial medicine. Proceedings of the 27th Annual Conference and Expo, Association of Avian Veterinarians. San Antonio (TX): 2006. p. 51–60.

35. La Regina MC, Lonigro J, Woods L, et al. Valvular endocarditis associated with experimental Erysipelothrix rhusiopathiae infection in the opossum (Didelphis virginiana). Lab Anim Sci 1988;38:159–61.

36. Lonigro JG, LaRegina MC. Characterization of Erysipelothrix rhusiopathiae isolated from an opossum (Didelphis virginiana) with septicemia. J Wildl Dis 1988;24:557–9.

37. Ruiz-Pina HA, Cruz-Reyes A. The opossum Didelphis virginiana as a synanthropic reservoir of Trypanosoma cruzi in Dzidzilche, Yucatan, Mexico. Mem Inst Oswaldo Cruz 2002;97:613–20.

38. Sherwood BF, Rowlands DT Jr, Hackel DB, et al. Bacterial endocarditis, glomerulonephritis and amyloidosis in the opossum (Didelphis virginiana). Am J Pathol 1968;53:115–26.

39. Sherwood BF, Rowlands DT Jr, Vakilzadeh J, et al. Experimental bacterial endocarditis in the opossum (Didelphis virginiana). 3. Comparison of spontaneously occurring endocarditis with that induced experimentally by pyogenic bacteria and fungi. Am J Pathol 1971;64:513–20.

40. Vakilzadeh J, Rowlands DT Jr, Sherwood BF, et al. Experimental bacterial endocarditis in the opossum (Didelphis virginiana). II. Induction of endocarditis with a single injection of Streptococcus viridans. J Infect Dis 1970;122:89–92.

41. Grollman A. Hypertension in the opossum Didelphis virginiana. Am J Physiol 1970;218:80–2.
42. Diters RW, Ryan MJ. Vegetative endocarditis with generalized bacterial embolism in association with phlegmon induced by Dracunculus insignis in a raccoon. Cornell Vet 1980;70:213–7.
43. Pietrzak SM, Pung OJ. Trypanosomiasis in raccoons from Georgia. J Wildl Dis 1998;34:132–6.
44. Ryan CP, Hughes PE, Howard EB. American trypanosomiasis (Chagas' disease) in a striped skunk. J Wildl Dis 1985;21:175–6.
45. Kocan AA. Parasitic diseases of wild mammals. In: Samuel WM, Pybus MJ, Kocan AA, editors. Parasitic diseases of wild mammals. Ames: Iowa State Press; 2001. p. 520–3.
46. Hobbs BA, Griffith JW. Cor pulmonale and cardiac failure in a skunk. J Am Vet Med Assoc 1984;185:1438–9.
47. Hwang YT, Wobeser G, Lariviere S, et al. Streptococcus equisimilis infection in striped skunks (Mephitis mephitis) in Saskatchewan. J Wildl Dis 2002;38:641–3.
48. Snyder DE, Hamir AN, Hanlon CA, et al. Dirofilaria immitis in a raccoon (Procyon lotor). J Wildl Dis 1989;25:130–1.
49. Christensen BM, Shelton ME. Laboratory observations on the insusceptibility of raccoons to Dirofilaria immitis. J Wildl Dis 1978;14:22–3.
50. Richardson DJ, Owen WB, Snyder DE. Helminth parasites of the raccoon (Procyon lotor) from north-central Arkansas. J Parasitol 1992;78:163–6.
51. Telford SR Jr, Forrester DJ. Hemoparasites of raccoons (Procyon lotor) in Florida. J Wildl Dis 1991;27:486–90.
52. Chu V, Otero JM, Lopez O, et al. Method for noninvasively recording electrocardiograms in conscious mice. BMC Physiol 2001;1:1–6.
53. Szabuniewicz JM, Szabuniewicz M. The electrocardiogram of the Virginia opossum (Didelphis virginiana). Zentralbl Veterinarmed A 1978;25:785–93.
54. Cieslar G, Sieron A, Rzepka E, et al. Normal electrocardiogram in guinea pig. Acta Physiol Pol 1986;37:139–49.
55. Brewer NR, Cruise LJ. Physiology. In: Manning PJ, Ringler DH, Newcomer CE, editors. Biology of the laboratory rabbit. 2nd edition. San Diego: Academic Press; 1994. p. 63–8.
56. Reusch B. Investigation and management of cardiovascular disease in rabbits. In practice 2005;27:418–25.
57. Bublot I, Randolph RW, Chalvet-Monfrey K, et al. The surface electrocardiogram in domestic ferrets. J Vet Cardiol 2006;8:87–93.
58. Francq E. Electrocardiogram of the opposum during feigned sleep. J Mammal 1970;51:395.
59. Hamlin RL, Hren J, Sparrow PV. Electrocardiographic evaluation of the healthy raccoon (Procyon lotor). Am J Vet Res 1986;47:814–7.
60. Silverman S, Tell L. Radiology of rodents, rabbits & ferrets. Elsevier: St Louis (MO); 2005.
61. Gabrische K, Grimm F, Isenbugel E, et al. Atlas of diagnostic radiology of exotic pets. Philadelphia: Saunders; 1991.
62. Stepien RL, Benson KG, Wenholz LJ. M-mode and Doppler echocardiographic findings in normal ferrets sedated with ketamine hydrochloride and midazolam. Vet Radiol Ultrasound 2000;41:452–6.
63. Vastenburg MH, Boroffka SA, Schoemaker NJ. Echocardiographic measurements in clinically healthy ferrets anesthetized with isoflurane. Vet Radiol Ultrasound 2004;45:228–32.
64. Stypmann J. Doppler ultrasound in mice. Echocardiography 2007;24:97–112.

65. Ivey E, Carpenter JW. Chapter 32: African hedgehogs. In: Quesenberry KE, Carpenter JW, editors. Ferrets, rabbits & rodents, clinical medicine and surgery. St. Louis (MO): Saunders; 2004. p. 339–53.
66. Rouleau J, Chuck L, Hollosi P, et al. Verapamil preserves cardiac contractility in the hereditary cardiomyopathy of the Syrian hamster. Circ Res 1982;50:405–12.
67. Watanabe M, Kawaguchi H, Onozuka H, et al. Chronic effects of enalapril and amlodipine on cardiac remodeling in cardiomyopathic hamster hearts. J Cardiovas Pharmacol 1998;32:248–59.
68. Delaney CJ. Special rodents: chinchillas. In: Delayney CJ, editor. Exotic companion medicine handbook. Lake Worth (FL): Zoological Education Network; 2000.
69. Carpenter JW. Exotic animal formulary. Philadelphia: Elsevier; 2001.
70. Yang XP, Liu YH, Rhaleb NE, et al. Echocardiographic assessment of cardiac function in conscious and anesthetized mice. Am J Physiol 1999;277:H1967–74.
71. Salemi VM, Bilate AM, Ramires FJ, et al. Reference values from M-mode and Doppler echocardiography for normal Syrian hamsters. Eur J Echocardiogr 2005;6:41–6.
72. Akula A, Kota MK, Gopisetty SG, et al. Biochemical, histological and echocardiographic changes during experimental cardiomyopathy in STZ-induced diabetic rats. Pharmacol Res 2003;48:429–35.
73. Cetin N, Cetin E, Toker M. Echocardiographic variables in healthy guinea pigs anaesthetized with ketamine-xylazine. Laboratory Animals 2004;39:100–6.
74. Lightfoot TL. Therapeutics of African pygmy hedgehogs and prairie dogs. Vet Clin North Am Exot Anim Pract 2000;3:155–72, vii.
75. Morrisey JK, Carpenter JW. Chapter 41: Formulary. In: Quesenberry KE, Carpenter JW, editors. Ferrets, rabbits & rodents, clinical medicine and surgery. St. Louis (MO): Saunders; 2004. p. 436–44.
76. Laber-Laird K, Swindle MM, Fleckness P. Handbook of rabbit and rodent medicine. Philadelphia: Elsevier; 1996.
77. van Steeg TJ, Freijer J, Danhof M, et al. Pharmacokinetic-pharmacodynamic modelling of S(-)-atenolol in rats: reduction of isoprenaline-induced tachycardia as a continuous pharmacodynamic endpoint. Br J Pharmacol 2007;151:356–66.
78. Bhattacharya S, Palmieri G, Bertorini T, et al. The effects of diltiazem on dystrophic hamsters. Muscle and nerve 1981;5:73–8.
79. Carceles M, Aleixandre F, Fuente T, et al. Effects of rolipram, pimobendan and zaprinast on ischaemia-induced dysrhythmias and on ventricular cyclic nucleotide content in the anaesthetized rat; 2002.
80. Kobayashi A, Yamashita T, Kaneko M, et al. Effects of verapamil on experimental cardiomyopathy in the Bio 14.5 Syrian hamster. J Am Coll Cardiol 1987;10:1128–38.

Ferret Cardiology

Robert A. Wagner, VMD

KEYWORDS

- Ferret • Cardiology • Cardiac disease • Cardiomyopathy
- Arrhythmias • Acquired valvular disease

Cardiac disease is common in pet ferrets (*Mustela putorius furo*).[1–5] It is reasonable to expect the full spectrum of cardiac diseases in ferrets found in small companion mammal practice. Dilated cardiomyopathy (DCM), arrhythmias, and acquired valvular disease are the most common heart diseases this author sees in practice. Congenital defects in heart development are seldom reported, but atrial septal defect and patent ductus arteriosus occur. A variety of inflammatory myocardial diseases, including Toxoplasmosis, Aleutian disease virus, and fungal and bacterial sepsis, are rarely diagnosed in practice. Neoplasia of the heart is rarely reported, with lymphosarcoma being most common. Pericardial fluid from chyle or neoplasia (lymphosarcoma) occurs with few reports in the literature. Nonbacterial thrombotic endocarditis is associated with myxomatous aortic valve degeneration.[6] Ferrets are definitive hosts for *Dirofilaria immitus,* and heartworm disease should be on the differential list in endemic areas.

CLINICAL PRESENTATION OF CARDIAC DISEASE

Clinical presentation of cardiac disease in the ferret ranges from an asymptomatic, incidental finding to fulminant heart failure.[1–4] Ferrets with clinical heart disease are generally weak, exercise intolerant, dyspneic, and often have pale or cyanotic mucus membranes with prolonged capillary refill time. Occasionally ferrets cough from pulmonary edema, heartworm infections, or main stem bronchi compression from an enlarged heart. Rear leg weakness can be seen and is thought to be associated with general weakness or from congestive heart failure (CHF). Left- and right-sided CHF can produce thoracic effusions, moist rales, ascites, or organomegaly. Respiratory rate may be increased, especially if thoracic effusions are present. Heart murmurs are common with DCM and valve insufficiency but are uncommon in hypertrophic cardiomyopathy (HCM). Clinicians may have difficulty determining the origin of heart murmurs. Often only a nonspecific left parasternal systolic murmur is heard. Holosystolic murmurs are most often caused by valvular regurgitation. Left apical murmurs are usually mitral valve, and right parasternal murmurs may be tricuspid valve insufficiency. Heart murmurs vary not only in location and duration but also in intensity.

Surgical Veterinary Services, Division of Laboratory Animal Resources, S1040 Biomedical Science Tower, University of Pittsburgh, PA 15261, USA
E-mail address: bwagner@pitt.edu

Vet Clin Exot Anim 12 (2009) 115–134
doi:10.1016/j.cvex.2008.09.001
1094-9194/08/$ – see front matter © 2009 Elsevier Inc. All rights reserved.

Anemia can cause low intensity variable location murmurs in ferrets because of low fluid viscosity. The normal heart rate is between 180 and 250 beats per minute (bpm). Sinus arrhythmia may produce a pronounced decrease in heart rate with occasional pauses auscultated; this should not be confused with pathologic bradycardia. Increased heart rate (> 250 bpm) and gallop rhythms (third and fourth heart sounds auscultated) are common with DCM and HCM, respectively. Tachyarrhythmias can be seen with either form of cardiomyopathy or acquired valvular disease. Arrhythmias caused by premature ventricular contractions or second- or third-degree heart blocks may be the only physical examination findings and should be evaluated thoroughly to determine their cause and significance. Sinus rhythm, sinus tachycardia, and bradycardia caused by second-degree heart block can be seen in normal ferrets, ferrets with asymptomatic cardiac disease, and ferrets with clinical cardiac disease.

RADIOGRAPHY

Radiography is useful in diagnosing cardiovascular disease in ferrets. It is the standard for determining cardiac size and CHF (pleural effusion, pulmonary venous engorgement, and pulmonary edema). The appearance of the normal ferret radiograph is similar to that of other carnivores. The ferret's thoracic cavity and trachea are relatively long. The normal ferret's trachea is parallel or bent slightly ventral starting around the fourth or fifth thoracic vertebra. The heart is between the sixth and eighth ribs. Occasionally on the lateral radiographic projection, the heart appears elevated ("floating heart") above the sternum, mimicking pneumothorax (**Fig. 1**). This may be a normal finding on a ferret radiograph, however.

Radiographic signs of heart disease include a large globose heart shadow, an elevated trachea, pleural effusion, and increased contact between the heart shadow and the diaphragm or sternum (**Fig. 2**). Other radiographic signs include pulmonary edema, pulmonary venous congestion, ascites, hepatomegaly, and splenomegaly. An enlarged heart shadow may indicate increased heart size, a mediastinal or cardiac mass, or pericardial effusion; echocardiography may be necessary to differentiate these lesions. Thoracic radiographs facilitate monitoring heart disease; the size of the heart and other thoracic changes become more pronounced as disease progresses.

The modified vertebral heart score (VHS) method measures the heart size in vertebral units (**Figs. 3 and 4**).[7] The right lateral view is preferred to detect and measure cardiac enlargement. The long axis of the heart is measured from the bottom of main stem

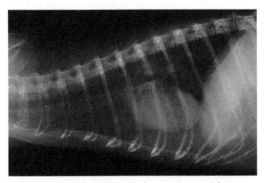

Fig. 1. Ferret lateral radiograph of thorax shows heart elevated form sternum. This "floating heart" has been seen in normal ferrets and in ferrets with cardiomyopathy and should be investigated further.

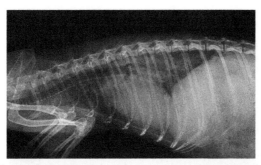

Fig. 2. Ferret lateral radiograph of thorax shows cardiomegaly and CHF. An elevated trachea, increased contact between the heart shadow, diaphragm, and sternum, pulmonary edema, and pulmonary venous congestion can be seen.

bronchus to the apex of the heart. The short axis is measured perpendicular to the long axis at the level of caudal vena cava. The length and width of the heart are registered as the number of vertebrae and estimated to the nearest one fourth of a vertebra. Long plus short axis equals VHS, which is recorded as the number of vertebrae starting at the cranial edge of the fifth thoracic vertebra (T5) to the caudal edge of the eighth thoracic vertebra (T8). Normal ferret VHS for the lateral view is 3.75 to 4.07 vertebrae. Clinicians should understand that VHS is not designed to diagnose cardiac disease but identify cardiomegaly (mainly secondary to volume overload). It is aimed more at reducing the rate of false-positive diagnoses but at the cost of more false-negative diagnoses. VHS does not improve the diagnosis of cardiac disease in dogs[8] and may apply similarly to ferrets.

The heart shadow size also can be compared with the number of rib spaces, with approximately 2.3 rib spaces being used as gauge for normal (**Figs. 3** and **4**). In right lateral position, the short axis of the cardiac silhouette is measured perpendicular to the long axis at the level of caudal vena cava. The mean intercostal space for ferrets is 2.28. The right lateral short axis intercostal space measurement is considered the best indicator of cardiomegaly and predictive of cardiac disease.[9] In cases of pleural

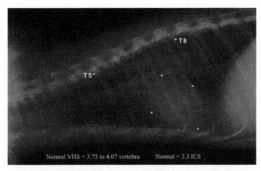

Fig. 3. Normal ferret lateral radiograph shows vertebral heart score (VHS) and intercostal space (ICS) determination of heart size. The long axis of the heart is measured from the bottom of main stem bronchus to the apex of the heart. The short axis is measured perpendicular to the long axis at the level of caudal vena cava. The length of the heart is recorded as the number of vertebrae, which starts at the cranial edge of the fifth thoracic vertebra. Long plus short axis = VHS.

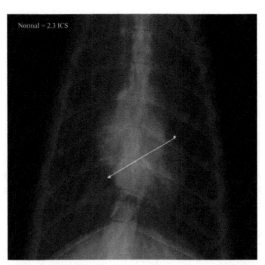

Fig. 4. Normal ferret ventrodorsal radiograph shows where to measure the heart for intercostal space determination. This heart is 2.1 intercostal space, consistent with a normal heart size.

effusion, thoracic fluid cytology should be performed to differentiate cancer, pyothorax, and chylothorax. Thoracic masses, which usually occur in the anterior mediastinum, are common in ferrets. Lymphosarcoma is the most common type of thoracic neoplasia in the ferret, but other cancers also occur.

Ascites, although less common than pleural effusion, is seen in later stages of CHF. Pulmonary venous congestion and pulmonary edema with a mixed interstitial and alveolar pattern containing air bronchograms is commonly seen in CHF. Hepatosplenomegaly may be seen with CHF, but noncardiac disease also must be considered.

Ultrasound is the method of choice for diagnosing structural and functional cardiac abnormalities. Pleural and pericardial effusions, heartworms, and mediastinal masses are readily identified with ultrasound. Echocardiography can be used to diagnose heartworms but may be of low sensitivity, and it requires good sonography skills. Heartworms appear as hyperechoic parallel bright lines within the right atria, ventricle, or pulmonary artery. Ultrasound is essential in differentiating DCM from HCM and tailoring treatment course. Standard M-mode measurements (**Tables 1** and **2; Fig. 5**) include chamber dimensions, wall thickness, and indices of systolic function.[10,11] Body weight does not affect M-mode measurements.[10] In DCM there is an increased left ventricular internal diameter in diastole and in systole (LVIDd and LVIDs). There is decreased fractional shortening (FS), and often the left atrium is dilated (left atrium appendage diameter). Less often the right ventricle is also dilated. HCM is characterized by gross thickening of the septum (IVSd and IVSs) and left ventricular free wall (LVWd and LVWs) and decreased left ventricular chamber dimensions (LVIDd and LVIDs). The walls of the left ventricle may be thickened symmetrically or asymmetrically. FS may be normal, increased, or slightly decreased with HCM in ferrets (**Fig. 6**). Acquired valvular disease is characterized by thickening and increased echogenicity of any of the valves in older ferrets. The mitral valve seems to be most commonly affected, but the actual frequency has not been reported. The diastolic dimension of the left ventricle is increased, but the systolic dimension is normal to slightly increased, which indicates normal myocardial contractility. This condition is caused by the permissive effect of the mitral valve regurgitation, which allows the ventricle to eject against low atrial

Table 1
Echocardiographic data from clinical healthy ferrets anesthetized with isoflurane

Parameter (n = 29)	Mean	SD	Range	Median
IVSd (mm)	3.4	0.4	2.5–4.4	3.4
IVSs (mm)	4.4	0.6	3.3–5.4	4.4
LVIDd (mm)	9.8	1.4	6.8–12.7	9.6
LVIDs (mm)	6.9	1.3	4.5–9.7	6.9
LVWd (mm)	2.7	0.5	1.8–3.7	2.7
LVWs (mm)	3.8	0.8	2.4–5.9	3.8
FS (%)	29.5	7.9	13.9–48.7	28.0
Ao (mm)	4.4	0.6	3.3–6.0	4.2
LAAD (mm)	5.8	0.9	3.2–7.3	5.7
LAAD/Ao	1.3	0.2	1.0–1.8	1.3
EPSS (mm)	1.2	0.6	0–2.2	1.2

Abbreviations: Ao, aorta diameter; EPSS, E-point to septal separation; FS, fractional shortening; IVSd and IVSs, thickness of the interventricular septum in diastole and systole; LAAD, left atrium appendage diameter; LVIDd and LVIDs, left ventricular internal diameter in diastole and systole; LVWd and LVWs, thickness of the left ventricular free wall in diastole and systole; SD, standard deviation.

Data from Maartje HAC, Vastenburg, Boroffka S, et al. Echocardiographic measurements in clinically healthy ferrets anesthetized with isoflurane. Vet Radiol Ultrasound 2004;45(3):228–32.

pressures while the aortic valve is closed. FS is normal to increased in acquired valvular disease because of low pressure regurgitation across atrioventricular valves. Tricuspid or mitral regurgitation is best demonstrated using Doppler (color flow or pulse wave) methods.

Dehydrated ferrets may have an increased diastolic left ventricular interventricular septum (IVSd) and free wall thickness that exceed normal limits. Dehydrated ferrets may have a decreased LVIDd and LVIDs, which can produce end-systolic cavity obliteration in ferrets. Altered hydration status may produce echocardiographic changes in ferrets—as seen in cats—that can lead to the erroneous diagnosis of cardiomyopathy.[12] Ferrets require little preparation for echocardiographic examination. Probes need to have a small footprint and be 7 to 10 MHz frequency. Image quality is often compromised by rib shadowing, rapid respiratory, and heart rates.

At times only a quick qualitative assessment of the ventricular contractility and wall thickness is all that can be observed in a ferret in CHF or in a difficult-to-restrain patient. Sedation is neither required nor desirable except in uncooperative patients. If sedation is used, the potential influence of the drug on heart rate, chamber dimensions, and ventricular motion must be considered in the interpretation. Ideally, hair is clipped over the left and right precordial transducer locations. Satisfactory images almost always can be obtained by parting the hair coat on the sides of the chest and by applying a liberal quantity of coupling gel or wetting the area with water or alcohol and then applying coupling gel. Ferrets may be examined in dorsal recumbency, scruffed (vertical), or laterally recumbent positions without substantial alteration of examination technique. The image quality is enhanced by positioning the animal in lateral recumbency on a table with an opening that allows transducer manipulation and examination from beneath the animal. This position results in the heart contacting a larger area of the lateral thorax and creates a larger ultrasound window for examination.

Electrocardiography (ECG) is used primarily to determine abnormal rhythms and electrical conduction/propagation disturbances. ECG data from four studies of

Table 2
Two-dimensional, M-mode, and Doppler echocardiographic values obtained normal adult ferrets sedated with ketamine and midazolam

Variable	N	Mean (SD)
Age (y)	30	2.3 (1.0)
Weight (kg)	30	1.17 (0.36)
HR (bpm)	29	273 (31)
IVSd (cm)	30	0.36 (0.07)
IVSs (cm)	30	0.48 (0.11)
LVIDd (cm)	30	0.88 (0.15)
LVIDs (cm)	30	0.59 (0.15)
LVWd (cm)	30	0.42 (0.11)
LVWs (cm)	30	0.58 (0.99)
FS (%)	30	33 (14)
EF (%)	27	69 (19)
RVWd (cm)	27	0.12 (0.03)
RVIDd (cm)	28	0.38 (0.10)
LA diameter (cm)	26	0.71 (0.18)
AO diameter (cm)	25	0.53 (0.10)
LA:AO	26	1.33 (0.27)
PA diameter (cm)	27	0.48 (0.9)
Doppler HR (bpm)	29	280 (32)
AO max (m/s)	25	0.89 (0.20)
AO VTI (cm)	25	5.15 (1.45)
AO CSA (cm^2)	25	0.23 (0.08)
AO SV (mL)	21	1.19 (0.60)
AO CO (mL/min)	21	330 (185)
AO CI (mL/min/kg)	21	261 (117)
PA max (m/s)	29	1.10 (0.14)
PA VTI (cm)	29	6.70 (1.05)
PA CSA (cm^2)	27	0.19 (0.06)
PA SV (mL)	27	1.22 (0.5)
PA CO (mL/min)	26	346 (145)
PA CI (mL/min/kg)	26	296 (124)
Mitral E (m/s)	15	0.70 (0.10)
Mitral A (m/s)	15	0.52 (0.11)
Mitral E:A	15	1.38 (0.32)

Measurements were obtained from 30 animals unless otherwise noted. Mean (standard deviation), median, first and third quartile values, and range are presented. Echocardiographic abbreviations are as noted in text.

Abbreviations: bpm, beats per minute; CSA, cross-sectional area; NA, not applicable.

Data from Stepien RL, Benson KG, Wenholz LJ. M-mode and Doppler echocardiographic findings in normal ferrets sedated with ketamine hydrochloride and midazolam. Vet Radiol Ultrasound 2000;41(5):452–6.

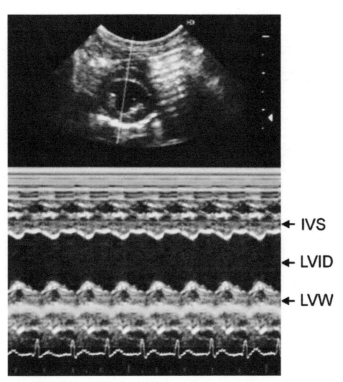

Fig. 5. Right parasternal short axis view and M-mode. tracing of the left ventricle, just below the mitral valve. IVS, interventricular septum; LVID, left ventricle internal diameter; LVW, left ventricular free wall. (*From* Maartje HAC, Vastenburg, Boroffka S, et al. Echocardiographic measurements in clinically healthy ferrets anesthetized with isoflurane. Vet Radiol Ultrasound 2004;45(3):229; with permission.)

clinically normal ferrets is presented in **Table 3**.[1,9,13,14] In one study, however, experimentally induced right ventricular hypertrophy and corresponding right mean electrical axis deviation in ferrets was not detected by ECG.[15] S-T segment elevation is seen in normal ferrets and in ferrets with cardiac disease. Other changes in the QRS-T complex are seen in normal ferrets and in ferrets with cardiac disease, but the significance of some of these changes remains unknown and needs to be studied. Generally the ferret ECG resembles the canine QRS complex (tall R waves) and the P waves are small, as in a cat (**Fig. 7**). Right lateral recumbency is the standard position for ECG recording. Sternal positioning changes mean electrical axis, P wave amplitude, R wave amplitude in leads I and II, and Q (or S) wave amplitude in lead I.[14] Often only a single lead (lead II) is needed to identify and characterize an arrhythmia. With cardiac disease, sinus tachycardia is the most common rhythm (**Fig. 8**); occasionally premature atrial contraction, premature ventricular contraction, and atrial fibrillation occur. Second- and third-degree heart (A-V) blocks are the most common conduction disturbances and can cause life-threatening bradycardia (**Figs. 9** and **10**). Severe bradycardia (< 80 bpm) carries a poor prognosis, and ferrets often die in 1 to 2 months of CHF when not treated. Ferrets with severe bradycardia can be treated with isoproterenol, metaproterenol, or an implantable pacemaker.[16,17] It seems that an intrinsic rate of 50 to 80 bpm must be treated to prevent progression to CHF. If a ferret with bradycardia is not weak, inactive, or in CHF there may be little improvement with treatment.

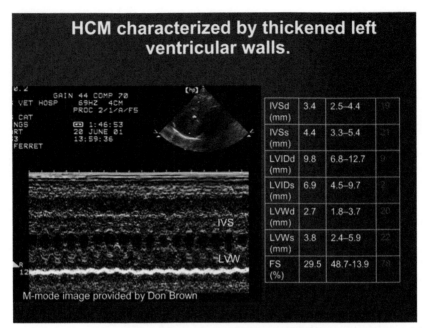

Fig. 6. Right parasternal short axis view and M-mode of HCM. Note the thickened left ventricle walls in systole and in diastole, the small LVIDs, and increased FS of 78%.

Table 3
Electrocardiographic data from clinically normal ferrets

	Fox[a]	Boonyapakorn[a]	Bone[a]	Bublot
Average age (mo)	5.2	—	—	—
Male: female ratio	1.25	—	—	—
Body weight (kg)	1.4 ± 0.2	—	—	—
Heart rate (beats/min)	233 ± 22	224 ± 51	196 ± 26.5	430 ± 250
Rhythm				
Normal sinus rhythm	0.67	—	—	—
Sinus arrhythmia	0.33	—	—	—
MEA (frontal plane)	77.22 ± 12	−10–104.5	64.84 ± 20.49	75 ± 100
Lead II				
P amplitude (mV)	0.122 ± 0.007	0.05–0.2	NA	≤ 0.2
P duration (s)	0.024 ± 0.004	0.02–0.04	NA	0.01 ± 0.03
PR interval (s)	0.047 ± 0.003	0.03–0.08	0.056 ± 0.009	0.03 ± 0.06
QRS duration (s)	0.043 ± 0.003	0.02–0.04	0.044 ± 0.008	0.02 ± 0.05
R amplitude (mV)	1.46 ± 0.84	0.5–2.7	2.21 ± 0.42	1 ± 2.8
QT interval (s)	0.12 ± 0.04	0.08–0.12	0.109 ± 0.018	0.06 ± 0.16

Abbreviation: NA, not available.
[a] Sedated with ketamine and xylazine.
Data from Refs.[1,10,14,15]

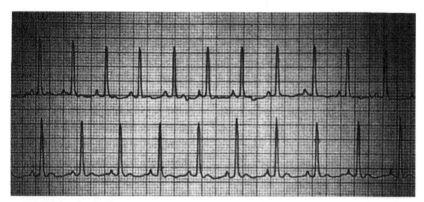

Fig. 7. Normal lead II ferret ECG. Small P waves, large R waves, and small to nonexistent Q or S waves characterize the normal P-QRS complex.

Ferrets with a second-degree heart block and presenting heart rates of 100 to 160 bpm may not warrant positive inotrope treatment (see **Fig. 10**) or pacemaker implantation.

OTHER DIAGNOSTIC TESTS

Heartworm-infected ferrets have low, transient concentrations of microfilaria, making microfilaria detecting tests unreliable. ELISA-based antigen tests (IDEXX Snap heartworm antigen test) have been shown to be effective 5 to 6 months after infection but may produce false-negative results because of low worm burdens. Adult worms may be detected by ultrasound as early as 5 months after infection in the cranial vena cava and right side of the heart. The small numbers of heartworms in these animals also necessitates the use of occult heartworm tests because of absent or low numbers of circulating microfilaria. DNA-based polymerase chain reaction assays are capable of sensitive and specific identification of the *Dirofilaria immitus* genetic material in blood specimens. Polymerase chain reaction assay is so sensitive that even a single heartworm cell can be detected, and it can be used for early detection of heartworm infection. This diagnostic approach to heartworm detection in ferrets needs to be further developed and validated.

Systolic blood pressure can be taken with Doppler and a pressure cuff using the digital branch of the tibial artery, the tail artery, or the pedal artery. This procedure is

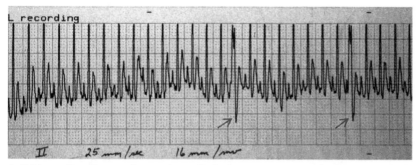

Fig. 8. With cardiac disease, sinus tachycardia is the most common rhythm seen. The heart rate is approximately 320 bpm, and occasional premature ventricular contractions (*arrows*) are seen in this case of DCM.

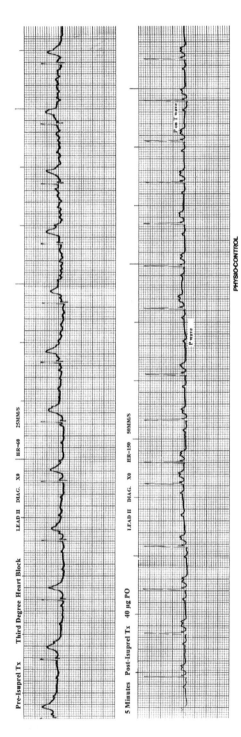

Fig. 9. Third-degree heart block in a ferret before and after Isuprel treatment. This ferret was weak and had CHF before treatment. It responded well to oral Isuprel by more than doubling its heart rate. (*From* Wagner RA. The treatment of third degree heart block in ferrets with subcutaneous or oral isoproterenol. Exotic DVM 2006;8(2):7; with permission.)

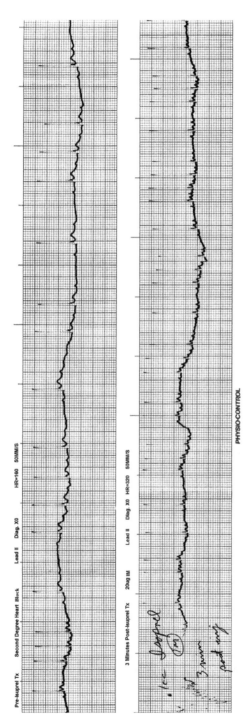

Fig. 10. Second-degree heart block in a ferret before and after Isuprel treatment. This ferret was quiet and alert before treatment. It responded well to intramuscular Isuprel by more than doubling its heart rate, but there was no corresponding increase in activity or clinical improvement. (*From* Wagner RA. The treatment of third degree heart block in ferrets with subcutaneous or oral isoproterenol. Exotic DVM 2006;8(2):7; with permission.)

difficult and usually performed under isoflurane anesthesia. Proper neonatal cuff selection is important. The cuff size should be approximately 40% of the circumference of the tarsus, carpus, tibia, or base of the tail. The smallest cuff available is a number 1 (infant size), which may be too large and may underestimate blood pressure. One study consistently underestimated indirect blood pressure measurements.[18] Normal direct systolic blood pressure ranges from 140 to 164 mm Hg and diastolic values range from 110 to 125 mm Hg depending on the reference used.[1,19,20] Direct blood pressure under urethane anesthesia is $140 \pm 35/110 \pm 31$ mm Hg.[19]

Cardiac biomarker serum cardiac troponin T is a sensitive and specific indicator of myocardial damage (doxorubicin cardiotoxicosis, traumatic injury, ischemia, and cardiac puncture) in the ferret. Reference range serum concentrations for normal ferrets (0.05–0.10 ng/mL) were at the detection limit of the assay, however, and a lack of clinical trials or controlled studies limits the clinical use of cardiac troponin T.[21] Natriuretic peptides have been studied in ferrets but are of limited clinical use to practitioners. Nonselective angiocardiography has been performed to exclude congenital cardiovascular lesions, diagnose heartworm disease, and better define cardiac chamber and great vessel size. This diagnostic modality primarily has been replaced with improved ultrasound techniques.

Cardiomyopathy is common in middle-aged and older domestic ferrets. DCM is most common but HCM is occasionally seen. An arrhythmogenic form of cardiomyopathy with little or no ventricular dilation or hypertrophy is probably a variant of DCM in which the conduction system is the primary site of degeneration and fibrosis. This arrhythmogenic form of cardiomyopathy often has normal myocardial function as determined by a normal FS and prevention or elimination of CHF with the use of positive chronotropes. Histologically, cardiomyopathies have myocyte degeneration, myofiber loss, and occasional inflammatory infiltrates, which eventually lead to fibrosis and myocardial dysfunction. Cardiomyopathies often progress to CHF. Most ferrets with cardiomyopathy have a good prognosis with proper diagnosis and treatment and may live a year or more from initial diagnosis. Ferrets with HCM have a poor prognosis, with sudden death and a survival expectation of only months after diagnosis.

The cause of cardiomyopathy is unknown or idiopathic in ferrets. In humans, cardiomyopathy may occur as a result of pre-existing endocrine diseases, viral disease, toxicities, and nutritional deficiency. In cats, DCM may be prevented and treated with the addition of taurine to the diet; in certain dog breeds, carnitine improves DCM. Similar dietary relationship may exist in ferrets, but this has not been proven. In humans, 40% of cases of DCM and most cases of HCM are thought to have a genetic origin.[22] Certain breeds of dogs have a genetic link to DCM, and the Maine Coon cat has a genetic basis for HCM. There is accumulating evidence in cats that most HCM is genetic in nature, with DNA coding aberrations for shortened telomeres and apoptosis of cardiomyocytes with minimal inflammation causing myocardial dysfunction (Bruce Williams, DACVP, personal communication, 2008). The inflammation seen may be the result of myofiber loss and not the cause. Idiopathic cardiomyopathy may have a similar genetic association in the ferret. Other known causes of cardiomyopathy in the ferret are limited, but in one ferret, cardiomyopathy was associated with a cryptococcal infection.

DCM is characterized by increased diastolic dimension of the left and right ventricles because of myocardial dysfunction. The normal afterload of systemic blood pressure does not allow normal end systolic emptying of the diseased ventricle so the ventricle remains dilated during and after systole. Indices of function, such as FS, are decreased and indices of heart size, such as end diastolic volume and end systolic volume, are increased. Ventricular wall thickness is decreased despite an increase in cardiac mass. The atria often dilate because of increased left ventricular filling pressure and decreased diastolic blood flow through the mitral valve; myocardial re-modeling occurs subsequent to the increased pressure and chamber dilation. In-creased atrial chamber workload promotes increased atrial chamber dilation and fatigue, which is an initiating factor in CHF. Left atrial chamber dilation and CHF are common consequence of DCM and valvular disease in ferrets. Lowering left ventric-ular filling pressure is essential for controlling CHF in humans, cats, and dogs. An S3 gallop is caused by the rapid filling of a dilated left ventricle (DCM or chronic volume overload in mitral valve disease). S3 is specific for an elevated left ventricular filling pressure and is highly predictive of CHF in humans.[23] Systolic heart murmurs and S3 gallop rhythm often improve with therapy in ferrets, which suggests that left ven-tricular filling pressure is lowered, averting CHF. In some cases, CHF is manifest as right-sided CHF with pleural effusion or as left-sided CHF with pulmonary edema. It is unclear which ferrets will develop each form of CHF, but both conditions are seen in clinical cases.

Hypertrophic cardiomyopathy in the ferret is a hyperplasia or thickening of individual muscle fibers of the heart, primarily the left ventricle. There is gross thickening of the septum and left ventricle free wall and decreased left ventricular dimensions. The heart size can be normal on radiographic projections with HCM, but chamber sizes of the heart decrease, reducing ventricular filling and cardiac output. These small chambers are apparent on ultrasound examination or at autopsy when the heart muscle is grossly sectioned (**Fig. 11**). Ultrasound is used to diagnose this form of cardiomyop-athy and formulate a treatment plan to increase ventricular filling and increase cardiac output. Because of the rarity of clinical cases of HCM and the presumed low preva-lence in ferrets, little is known about effective therapy of this condition either before or after the onset of CHF.

Treatment is aimed at improving diastolic filling of the ventricles and eliminating CHF if present. Beta blockers slow the heart rate and calcium channel blockers vasodilate coronary arteries, which increases myocardial perfusion and reduces heart rate and blood pressure. This combination of drug effects reduces myocardial oxygen con-sumption and increases cardiac output. Cardiac output and coronary flow (myocardial oxygen supply) must meet oxygen demand or anaerobic conditions prevail. An anaer-obic myocardium results in reduced contractility and dysrhythmias commonly seen in HCM. Diuretics and angiotensin-converting enzyme inhibitors are used for treating

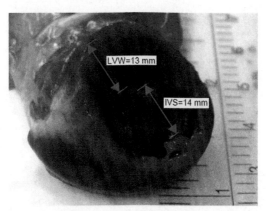

Fig. 11. Cross-section of hypertrophic left ventricle ferret heart. Severe hypertrophy of the IVS (14 mm) (2.5–5.4 mm) and the LVW (13 mm) (1.8–5.9 mm) produced few clinical signs. This ferret presented with a sudden onset of CHF and then died.

CHF. Aspirin or heparin therapy is not needed because arterial thromboemboli—as seen in cats with HCM—are rarely seen in ferrets.

Acquired valvular disease is the second most common heart disease seen in ferrets. Valvular endocardiosis is a degenerative change of unknown cause that affects the subendocardial valve leaflets and chordae tendineae in the middle aged to elderly ferret. Endocardiosis leads to progressive valvular incompetency with regurgitation of blood across the closed valve and eventually CHF. There is no reported incidence of which valves are most affected, but the mitral valve is probably affected most often, with the tricuspid valve and aortic valve less frequently involved. Gross lesions of advanced endocardiosis include opaque nodular thickening and shortening at the free edge and base of the valve leaflets. Mitral regurgitation leads to secondary dilatation of the left atrium and left ventricle, with the left atrium often being larger than the left ventricle. As cardiac failure progresses, left-sided CHF produces pulmonary edema and pleural effusion. The right ventricle may be dilated from tricuspid regurgitation and can progress to right-sided CHF, hepatosplenomegaly, and ascites.

The primary differential diagnosis of chronic valvular heart disease in ferrets is DCM. Ultrasound evaluation is essential to distinguish between the two disease entities based on the determination of any affected valves and ventricular contractility. Echocardiographic findings consistent with chronic valvular disease include cardiomegaly, thickened atrioventricular valves, and increased or normal FS with normal ventricular contractility (**Figs. 12** and **13**). An increased FS distinguishes this condition from DCM in which FS is often decreased. Valvular regurgitation is detected with color flow Doppler and pulse wave Doppler (**Figs. 14** and **15**). The regurgitant jet is generally large and often eccentric in ferrets with valvular disease and is less impressive and central in cases of DCM, in which it is caused by a mild distraction of the mitral valve cusps and mitral annular dilation rather than primary valvular pathology. Small regurgitant jets of blood through the mitral, aortic, pulmonic, and tricuspid valves occur in clinically healthy ferrets and should not be mistaken as cardiac pathology during ultrasound examination.

Metabolic disturbances often secondary to neoplasia can manifest as cardiovascular disease. Hypoglycemia caused by insulinoma, liver disease, or fasting can cause

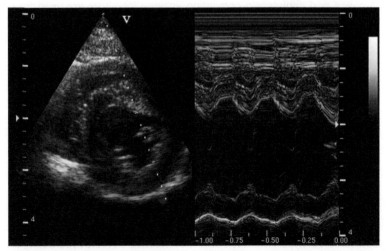

Fig. 12. Acquired valvular disease M-mode shows increased LVIDd = 18 mm (< 13 mm) causing cardiomegaly and normal to slightly increased FS = 46% (13.9%–48.7%).

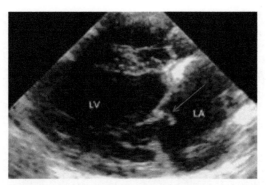

Fig. 13. Mitral valve thickening (*arrow*) seen in a ferret with chronic valvular disease.

bradycardia in ferrets. Functional pheochromocytomas can cause sinus tachycardia, hypertension, and weakness. Antemortem diagnosis of pheochromocytoma may be difficult to differentiate from primary cardiovascular disease. Determination of blood pressure, ultrasound examination of the chest and abdomen, and determination of urine or plasma catecholamine levels can help differentiate these diseases (**Table 4**). Hypoadrenalcorticism (Addison's disease) occasionally occurs in ferrets after bilateral adrenalectomy and results in hypotension- and hyperkalemia-induced cardiac arrhythmias. Hypothermia from renal failure, toxins, or cold exposure can cause severe bradycardia and heart block.

Heartworm disease in ferrets[2,5,24,25] is uncommon or possibly underdiagnosed, but more cases are being reported in heartworm-endemic areas, especially in ferrets kept outdoors. Ferrets in heartworm-endemic areas should be maintained on monthly heartworm prevention. Because of the small size of the ferret heart, as few as two heartworms may result in fatal cardiac insufficiency. If heartworms are present in the right ventricle or pulmonary artery at necropsy in any ferret, this was the likely cause of death.

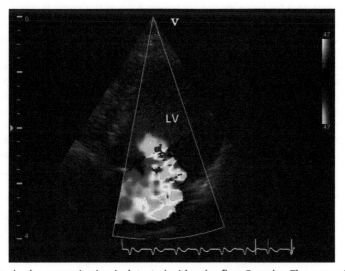

Fig. 14. Mitral valve regurgitation is detected with color flow Doppler. The regurgitant jet is large and eccentric, as is seen in most cases of acquired valvular disease.

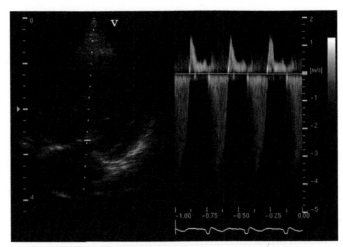

Fig. 15. Mitral valve regurgitation is detected with pulse wave Doppler.

Clinical signs of heartworm disease in the ferret are similar to those in the dog but they progress more rapidly, so early diagnosis is important. Clinical signs may include coughing, dyspnea, tachypnea, anorexia, pulmonary rales, holosystolic heart murmur, ascites, pleural effusion, and sometimes sudden death. Eosinophilia is not a common finding in ferret heartworm disease, but monocytosis, bilirubinuria, and hypochloremia have been reported.[5] Radiographic changes consist of pleural effusion and tortuous, dilated pulmonary vasculature. Sonographic examination often shows enlarged dilated right atrium and ventricle and tricuspid regurgitation. Clinical heartworm disease in ferrets presents similarly to other cardiac disease and must be considered especially in endemic areas.

CARDIAC THERAPEUTIC AGENTS FOR FERRETS

In general, treatment for heart disease in ferrets follows the same therapeutic guidelines used in dogs and cats. Pharmacokinetic studies have not been conducted for cardiovascular drugs in ferrets; scaling down doses already in use for cats works well clinically (**Table 5**).[26]

Furosemide (Lasix) at 2 to 3 mg/kg intramuscularly or intravenously (IV) every 8 to 12 hours is used initially for ferrets in fulminant myocardial failure and at 1 to 2 mg/kg orally every 12 hours for long-term maintenance therapy. Hypokalemia with long-term therapy is rarely a problem. Abdominocentesis or thoracocentesis can be effective at maintaining some CHF cases long-term. Vasodilators are an important part of cardiac therapy. Nitroglycerin 2% cream is a venous dilator that can be used at one-sixteenth to one-eighth in inside the pinna for the first 24 hours in emergencies.

Table 4		
Normal plasma and urine catecholamine concentrations in ferrets		
	Plasma (pg/m) $n = 5$	Urine (mg/g Creatinine) $n = 4$
Norepinephrine	159	53.3
Epinephrine	64	28.2
Dopamine	62.8	5.5

From RA Wagner, VMD, unpublished data, 2003.

Table 5
Drug doses, route, and indications for cardiac diseases in the ferret

Drug	Dose	Route	Indication
Atenolol	3–6 mg/kg every 24 h	Oral	HCM
Atropine	0.02–0.04 mg/kg	Subcutaneous or intramuscular	Bradyarrythmias
Digoxin pediatric elixir (Lanoxin)	0.005–0.01 mg/kg every 24 h	Oral	Superventricular tachyarrhythmia or DCM
Diltiazem	1.5–7.5 mg/kg every 12 h	Oral	HCM
Dobutamine	5–10 μg/kg/min	IV slow infusion	Used to treat acute fulminant CHF
Enlapril (Enacard, Vasotec)	0.25–0.5 mg/kg every 48 h	Oral	CHF
Furosemide (Lasix)	2–3 mg/kg every 8–12 h 1–2 mg/kg every 8–12 h	Intramuscular/IV Oral	Fulminant pulmonary edema Long-term CHF maintenance therapy
Isoproterenol (Isuprel)	40–50 μg/kg every 12 h 20–25 μg/kg every 4–6 h	Oral Intramuscular or subcutaneous	Third-degree heart block
Ivermectin	0.02 mg/kg	Oral or subcutaneous	Heart worm prevention
Ivermectin	50 μg/kg every 30 d	Subcutaneous	Heart worm treatment
Melarsomine	2.5 mg/kg at 1, 30, & 31 d	Intramuscular	Heart worm treatment
Metaproterenol (Alupent)	0.25–0.5 to 1.0 mg/kg every 12 h	Oral	Third-degree heart block
Moxidectin (ProHeart)	0.1 mL (single dose)	Subcutaneous	Adulticide (heart worm); every 6 mo as preventone
Nitroglycerin	2% cream	Topical, 1/16–1/8 in area inside the pinna	CHF emergencies
Pimobendan (Vetmedin)	0.5 mg/kg every 12 h	Oral	DCM or mitral valve disease

Enalapril (Enacard, Vasotec) is an angiotensin-converting enzyme inhibitor used at 0.25 to 0.5 mg/kg orally every 48 hours initially and then can be increased to once-daily dosing if tolerated.

Hypotension is a common problem with angiotensin-converting enzyme inhibitors, and doses must be titrated for each ferret, especially in animals with renal compromise or dehydration. Currently, no evidence supports the preferential use of any angiotensin-converting enzyme inhibitor based on efficacy or safety in ferrets. Digoxin pediatric elixir (Lanoxin) works well in ferrets with superventricular tachyarrhythmia or DCM (0.005–0.01 mg/kg every 24 hours initial dose, then gradually increased to every 12 hours as needed). Therapeutic serum concentrations of 1 to 2 ng/mL should occur

10 to 12 hours after oral administration. Pimobendan (Vetmedin 0.5 mg/kg orally twice a day) is a positive inotropic and vasodilator that is safe and effective in cases of DCM or mitral valve disease. It increases ventricular contractility and reduces preload and afterload. Beta-blockers such as atenolol (3–6 mg/kg orally every 24 hours) or calcium channel blockers such as diltiazem (1.5–7.5 mg/kg orally every 12 hours) can reduce the heart rate in cases of HCM. Atropine (0.02–0.04 mg/kg subcutaneously or intramuscularly) is indicated to control bradyarrhythmias. Metaproterenol (Alupent 0.25–0.5–1.0 mg/kg orally twice a day) or isoproterenol (Isuprel 40–50 µg orally or 20–25 µg intramuscularly or subcutaneously per ferret every 4–6 hours) can be used to control third-degree heart block. Metaproterenol is more convenient than isoproterenol because of the longer duration of action but is not as effective at maintaining heart rates of more than 80 bpm. Isoproterenol can produce infarct-like myocardial necrosis, but this side effect has not been seen in the limited number of ferrets treated.[27]

Pacemaker implantation is an option for treating third-degree atrioventricular block. Ivermectin at 0.02 mg/kg orally or subcutaneously monthly is used to prevent maturation of third-stage heartworm larval development. Approved cat and dog heartworm preventive medications (selamectin, ivermectin, moxidectin, milbemycin oxime) have been used safely in ferrets. Adulticides such as melarsomine can produce severe reactions, including death, and should be used with caution. A single dose of moxidectin (ProHeart) at 0.1 mL subcutaneously per ferret has been used effectively and safely as an adulticide. Moxidectin at the same dose every 6 months can be used as a preventive for heartworm infection. Adjust doses for each individual cardiac case.

SUMMARY

The clinician must recognize that ferrets have only a few common cardiovascular diseases and often have concurrent diseases.[26] When presented with a suspicious cardiovascular case, an initial assessment needs to be made to differentiate cardiovascular disease from pulmonary disease, space-occupying lesions (tumors or fluid), heartworm infection, or metabolic disturbance. It is not always easy to make this distinction, and a minimum database may be necessary to arrive at a preliminary diagnosis. A thorough physical examination and chest radiographs are standard for diagnosing CHF. This approach often determines if a patient needs immediate stabilization and guides the initial therapeutic course. Once the patient is stable, additional diagnostics should be perused. If fluid is present in the chest or abdomen, an aspirate and cytology are needed to rule out cancer and decrease respiratory distress (thoracocentesis). An ECG should be done if an arrhythmia is present, and an ultrasound examination is essential for differentiating HCM from DCM and acquired valvular disease. Information that each of these steps yields is important for making the correct diagnosis, formulating a treatment plan, and determining a prognosis.

REFERENCES

1. Fox JG. Other systemic diseases. In: Fox JG, editor. Biology and diseases of the ferret. 2nd edition. Philadelphia: Lea & Febiger; 1998. p. 104, 203–6, 313–8.
2. Hoefer HL. Heart disease in ferrets. In: Bonagura JD, editor. Kirk's current veterinary therapy XIII: small animal practice. Philadelphia: WB Saunders Co.; 2000. p. 1144–8.
3. Petrie JP. Part I cardiac disease. In: Quesenberry KE, Carpenter JW, editors. Ferrets, rabbits, and rodents: clinical medicine and surgery. 2nd edition. Philadelphia: WB Saunders; 2004. p. 58–71.

4. Lewington JH. Cardiovascular disease. In: Ferret husbandry, medicine, and surgery. 2nd edition. Oxford (MA): Butterworth-Heinemann; 2007. p. 275–84.
5. Antinoff N. Clinical observations in ferrets with naturally occurring heartworm disease and preliminary evaluation of treatment with ivermection with and without melarsomine. Recent Adv Heartworm Dis 2002;45–7.
6. Kottwitz JJ, Luis-Fuentes V, Micheal B. Nonbacterial thrombotic endocarditis in a ferret (Mustela putorius furo). J Zoo Wildl Med 2006;37(2):197–201.
7. Stepien RL, Benson KG, Forrest LJ. Radiographic measurement of cardiac size in normal ferrets. Vet Radiol Ultrasound 1999;40(6):606–10.
8. Lamb CR, Tyler M, Boswood A, et al. Assessment of the value of the vertebral heart scale in the radiographic diagnosis of cardiac disease in dogs. Vet Rec 2000;146(24):687–90.
9. Boonyapakorn C. Cardiologic examinations in ferrets with and without heart disease [doctoral thesis]. Berlin: Freien Universität; 2007.
10. Maartje HAC, Vastenburg, Boroffka S, et al. Echocardiographic measurements in clinically healthy ferrets anesthetized with isoflurane. Vet Radiol Ultrasound 2004; 45(3):228–32.
11. Stepien RL, Benson KG, Wenholz LJ. M-mode and Doppler echocardiographic findings in normal ferrets sedated with ketamine hydrochloride and midazolam. Vet Radiol Ultrasound 2000;41(5):452–6.
12. Campbell FE, Kittleson MD. The effect of hydration status on the echocardiographic measurements of normal cats. J Vet Intern Med 2007;21(5):1008–15.
13. Bone L, Battles AH, Goldfarb RD, et al. Electrocardiographic values from clinically normal, anesthetized ferrets (Mustela putorius furo). Am J Vet Res 1988; 49(11):1884–7.
14. Bublot I, Randolph W, Chalvet-Monfray K, et al. The surface electrocardiogram in domestic ferrets. J Vet Cardiol 2006;8(2):87–93.
15. Smith SH, Bishop SP. The electrocardiogram of normal ferrets and ferrets with right ventricular hypertrophy. Lab Anim Sci 1985;35(3):268–71.
16. Wagner RA. The treatment of third degree heart block in ferrets with subcutaneous or oral isoproterenol. Exotic DVM 2006;8(2):6–7.
17. Sanchez-Migallon Guzman D, Mayer J, Melidone R, et al. Pacemaker implantation in a ferret (Mustela putorius furo) with third-degree atrioventricular block. Vet Clin North Am Exot Anim Pract 2006;9(3):677–87.
18. Olin JM, Smith TJ, Talcott MR. Evaluation of noninvasive monitoring techniques in domestic ferrets (Mustela putorius furo). Am J Vet Res 1997;58(10):1065–9.
19. Andrews PL, Bower AJ, Illman O. Some aspects of the physiology and anatomy of the cardiovascular system of the ferret, Mustela putorius furo. Lab Anim 1979; 13(3):215–20.
20. Kempf JE, Chang HT. The cardiac output and circulation time of ferrets. Proc Soc Exp Biol Med 1949;72(3):711–4.
21. O'Brien PJ, Dameron GW, Beck ML, et al. Cardiac troponin T is a sensitive, specific biomarker of cardiac injury in laboratory animals. Lab Anim Sci 1997;47(5):486–95.
22. Grunig E, Tasman JA, Kucherer H, et al. Frequency and phenotypes of familial dilated cardiomyopathy. J Am Coll Cardiol 1998;31:186–94.
23. Marcus GM, Gerber IL, McKeown H, et al. Association between phonocardiographic third and fourth heart sounds and objective measures of left ventricular function. JAMA 2005;293(18):2238–44.
24. McCall JW. Dirofilariasis in the domestic ferret. Clin Tech Small Anim Pract 1998; 13(2):109–12.

25. Heatley JJ. Small exotic mammal cardiovascular disease. In: Bergman, E, editor. Proceedings of the 28th Annual AAV Conference and Expo with the Association of Exotic Mammal Veterinarians. Boca Raton (FL): Association of Avian Veterinarians. 69.
26. Heatley JJ. Ferret cardiomyopathy. Compendium's standards of care emergency and critical care medicine 2007;8(3):7–11.
27. Rona G. Catecholamine cardiotoxicity. J Mol Cell Cardiol 1985;17(4):291–306.

Cardiovascular Physiology and Diseases of the Rabbit

Romain Pariaut, DVM, DACVIM–Cardiology, ECVIM-CA–Cardiology

KEYWORDS

- Cardiology • Congestive heart failure • Lagomorph
- Electrocardiography • Echocardiography • Arrhythmias

The domestic rabbit *(Oryctolagus cuniculus)* has been extensively used as an animal model for cardiovascular research. This model has allowed major advances in the study of atherosclerosis because it develops hypercholesterolemia and associated vascular lesions when fed a fat-enriched diet.[1] Conversely, little is known about the incidence, diagnosis, and treatment of cardiovascular diseases in the pet rabbit. Moreover, experimental models do not reproduce naturally occurring diseases of the rabbit and do not provide information applicable to the management of the house rabbit with cardiac disease. In this article, cardiac disease of the pet rabbit will be discussed with an emphasis on anatomic and physiologic features, physical examination, diagnostic tests, disease processes, and treatments.

CARDIOVASCULAR ANATOMY AND PHYSIOLOGY

The heart is the muscular pump of the cardiovascular system. It is the largest organ within the mediastinum, but represents only 0.20% of the pet rabbit body weight, in contrast to 0.76% of the dog's body weight, or other lagomorphs that are endurance runners *(Lepus* spp, *Sylvilagus* spp).[2] The heart and great vessels are surrounded by lung tissue. The cranial, middle, and accessory lobes surrounding the heart form a well-defined pocket, the cardiac fossa. In many cursorial lagomorphs, such as *Lepus* spp, an extended right cranial lobe is interposed between the sternum and the heart to cushion and provide protection to the heart. This feature is lacking in *Oryctolagus* spp, possibly as a result of domestication.[3] Rabbits have a left cranial vena cava in addition to the right cranial vena cava. This vessel terminates in a large coronary sinus that also drains the cardiac veins.[4] The right atrium receives deoxygenated blood from the two cranial and the caudal venae cavae. Once in the atrium, deoxygenated blood flows to the right ventricle through the right atrioventricular valve or tricuspid valve. The tricuspid valve, composed of only two cusps, is often described as a distinctive attribute of

Department of Clinical Sciences, School of Veterinary Medicine, Skip Bertman Drive, Louisiana State University, Baton Rouge, LA 70803, USA
E-mail address: rpariaut@vetmed.lsu.edu

Vet Clin Exot Anim 12 (2009) 135–144
doi:10.1016/j.cvex.2008.08.004
1094-9194/08/$ – see front matter © 2009 Elsevier Inc. All rights reserved.

vetexotic.theclinics.com

the rabbit. However, this feature is shared by many species, including the dog and the cat.[5,6] The right ventricle ejects blood into the lungs to be oxygenated. The newly oxygenated blood flows out of the lungs and into the left atrium through the pulmonary veins. From the left atrium, blood flows into the left ventricle and into the aorta to be distributed to the rest of the body. The left and right auricles are proportionally large compared with the body of the atria. In the rabbit heart, the conduction system is organized in a pattern similar to that of the dog and humans. There are a sinus node, internodal pathways, an atrioventricular node, a His bundle, and a left and right bundle branches.[4] The normal heart rate of the rabbit, when recorded by telemetry without any restraint, is approximately 220 beats/min.[7] Higher heart rates should be expected upon auscultation because of increased sympathetic tone secondary to stress. A healthy rabbit can have a heart rate between 200 and 300 beats/min.

Perhaps a consequence of domestication, the lungs of the rabbit are relatively smaller than those predicted for its body mass. They are lobulated into a cranial, middle, and caudal lung lobe on the right side; a cranial and caudal lung lobe on the left side; and an accessory lobe between the heart and the diaphragm. Twelve pairs of ribs form a small thoracic cavity comparatively to the body size. The diaphragm is the only muscle that significantly contributes to breathing.[3] These features may explain the high incidence of respiratory failure secondary to respiratory diseases and congestive heart failure in the rabbit. The rabbit has a physiologic respiratory rate of 30 to 60 breaths/min, which can increase significantly with stress.[8]

PHYSICAL EXAMINATION OF THE CARDIOVASCULAR SYSTEM
Restraint and Sedation

Because of its timid personality, its high sensitivity to stress, and the risk of self-induced injuries, the rabbit must be restrained carefully. The rabbit is also light sensitive, as it is a crepuscular animal, most active at dawn and dusk in the wild. To prevent excessive stress that may result in the aggravation of clinical signs or an erroneous interpretation of physical examination findings, the rabbit is examined in a quiet room and external stimuli are decreased by covering his eyes with a towel. Most of the cardiovascular work-up should be done with an assistant, who gently restrains the animal on a table covered with a nonslip surface.[9] The rabbit is maintained in sternal recumbency for the duration of the examination. Sedation may be required to prevent excessive stress and the risk of self-injury. Midazolam at a dose of 0.5 to 1.0 mg/kg given intramuscularly or intravenously gives satisfactory results, and has limited effects on the cardiovascular system.[8]

Signalment

Predisposition of the rabbit to acquired cardiovascular diseases is unknown, but their incidence increases with age. Hypertension secondary to renal disease, obesity, and hypercholesterolemia from an incorrect diet may increase the incidence of cardiac diseases.

Physical Examination

The rabbit should be first evaluated in its transport carrier to assess its behavior at rest and its respiratory rate. Examination of the cardiovascular system includes the evaluation of mucous membranes, capillary refill time, and peripheral arterial pulse, as well as thoracic and cardiac auscultation. Normal mucous membrane color is light pink. It is assessed by inspection of the oral and conjunctival mucous membranes.[10] Pale mucous membranes indicate decreased cardiac output and peripheral perfusion in a rabbit with normal packed cell volume. Dry gums reflect dehydration. Cyanosis is better assessed by examination of the tongue, and reflects hypoxemia. The capillary refill time is measured by applying digital pressure on the gums, releasing the pressure, and measuring the time it takes for the color to return.[11] Normal capillary refill time is less than 2 seconds. It is prolonged with decreased cardiac output. The central artery of the ear is easily accessible for palpation of the peripheral pulse. It provides information on the rate and regularity of the heartbeats. Its strength is an indicator of peripheral perfusion.

Thoracic auscultation and cardiac auscultation are best performed with a pediatric stethoscope. Because of the small size of the patient and its rapid respiratory and heart rates, only limited information can be gathered from auscultation. Respiratory and cardiac sounds are muffled in the presence of pleural effusion, but they may also be decreased in intensity if a large amount of subcutaneous and intrathoracic fat is present. Pulmonary edema results in increased bronchovesicular sounds and crackles. While crackles are best heard at the end of a forced inspiration, most rabbits with congestive heart failure present with rapid and superficial respiration. Therefore, the absence of crackles does not rule out pulmonary edema in the rabbit.[11]

Normal heart sounds are high frequency and best heard with the diaphragm of the stethoscope. As rabbits are obligate nose breathers, one should not manually occlude the nares to attenuate lung sounds during cardiac auscultation, as is commonly done in dogs.[10] Two heart sounds are normally musculted. The first heart sound occurs at the onset of systole and is associated with closure of the atrioventricular valves. The second heart sound corresponds to closure of the pulmonic and aortic valves. In the presence of severe structural cardiac disease, a third heart sound can be heard, resulting in a gallop rhythm. This third heart sound is generated during diastole and reflects impaired filling of a stiffened, noncompliant ventricle, or rapid filling of a dilated left ventricle.[11] Arrhythmias are usually first detected on auscultation, however this finding should always be confirmed with an electrocardiogram. Murmurs are generated by turbulent blood flow. In the rabbit, murmurs are usually systolic, mild to moderate in intensity, and heard best on the left or right sternal border. Because of the small size of the heart, it is almost impossible to precisely localize a murmur. There is a risk to overdiagnosing cardiac murmurs: excessive pressure of the stethoscope on the rabbit's compliant thoracic wall may cause partial obstruction of the right ventricular outflow tract creating a nonpathologic heart murmur. Moreover, respiratory sounds can mimic heart murmurs when the increased respiratory rate approximates the heart rate. As a result, an echocardiogram is indicated whenever a murmur is audible in a rabbit.

DIAGNOSTIC TESTS
Thoracic Radiographs

Survey radiographs reveal an astonishingly small chest in comparison to the size of the trunk. As a result, interpretation of cardiac and lung abnormalities can be challenging. It is facilitated by the use of digital radiography, which allows magnification of selected areas of the image on a high-definition monitor. On a lateral view, the cranial border of the heart is usually indistinguishable from the tissue opacity in the cranial mediastinum, which comprises the thymus and intrathoracic fat, and is usually superimposed with the front legs. The cardiac silhouette extends from the second rib to the caudal border of the fifth rib, or from the third to the sixth ribs. Obese rabbits may have a markedly enlarged cardiac silhouette secondary to the accumulation of pericardial fat. Generalized cardiomegaly is consistent with cardiac chamber dilation or hypertrophy, pericardial effusion, or the presence of a cardiac mass. The lung fields may be difficult to assess because of the small size of the thorax, and the difficulty of obtaining images in full inspiration. The veterinarian not familiar with thoracic radiographs of the rabbit may find it helpful to keep a set of chest films from a healthy rabbit and reference them to compare with radiographs of a rabbit with possible cardiac disease.

Electrocardiography

The electrocardiogram is usually recorded with the patient gently restrained in sternal recumbency (**Fig. 1**A). Because of rapid heart rate and small size of the atrial and ventricular complexes, interpretation is easier if the electrocardiogram is recorded at a speed of 50 mm/sec and an amplitude of 2 cm/mV. The normal cardiac activity is recorded on the surface electrocardiogram as a positive P wave followed by an upright QRS complex in lead II. The T wave is usually positive and reflects ventricular repolarization (see **Fig. 1**B).[10] The electrocardiogram should mostly be used for the diagnosis of arrhythmias when an irregular rhythm is detected on auscultation. Because little is known about the electrocardiographic changes associated with cardiac diseases in the rabbit, the use of P wave and QRS complex changes in morphology to assess cardiac chamber dilation or hypertrophy is not recommended (**Table 1**).

Blood Pressure Measurement

Indirect blood pressure measurement is usually obtained by the Doppler technique. A small cuff, with a width equal to 30% to 40% of the limb circumference is placed on a front leg proximal to the elbow. The Doppler crystal is covered with coupling gel and placed on the palmar surface, proximal to the carpus. The cuff is inflated, and then slowly deflated until the signal returns. The systolic pressure is measured with this technique. Normal blood pressure in the rabbit is known from telemetry recordings. Blood pressure and heart rate tend to increase in the rabbit during the night. Systolic blood pressure recorded by telemetry varies between 93 and 99 mm Hg.[12] Most commonly, systolic blood pressure measured with the Doppler technique in the hospital environment is between 120 and 180 mm Hg.

Echocardiography

Echocardiography gives valuable information about chamber dimensions, left ventricular function, the presence of abnormal communications between cardiac chambers or vessels, and blood flow. The hair may have to be clipped at the transducer site, but most of the time good-quality images can be obtained by simply wetting the site with alcohol, parting the hair coat on either side, and then applying coupling gel. Usually the

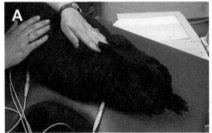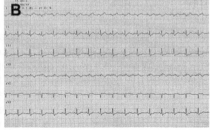

Fig.1. (A) Electrocardiographic recording in a rabbit. (B) Normal 6-lead electrocardiogram in a rabbit. Speed 50 mm/s, amplitude 20 mm/mV.

Table 1
Values for electrocardiographic variables from five normal pet rabbits with a mean heart rate of 240 beats/min

Electrocardiographic Variable	Value
P wave amplitude	0.04–0.07 mV
P wave duration	20–40 ms
R wave amplitude	0.12–0.2 mV
QRS duration	30–40 ms
P-R interval	50–70 ms

From Romain Pariaut, unpublished data, 2007.

rabbit is held in sternal recumbency on a padded table, with its thorax placed above an opening in the table, which allows transducer manipulation and examination from beneath the animal (**Fig. 2**). The transducer is placed first on the right sternal border between the fourth and sixth intercostal space, where the precordial impulse can be palpated. The views classically described in dogs and cats can be obtained in the rabbit. Precise measurements are not necessary, and valuable information is gathered by subjective assessment of the size and function of the four cardiac chambers on two-dimensional images. Similar to most mammals, the left atrial diameter is 1.0 to 1.5 times the diameter of the aorta, left and right atria are comparable in size, the aorta and the main pulmonary artery have the same diameter, and the left ventricular free wall thickness is similar to the interventricular septum thickness. The thickness of right ventricular free wall and the diameter of the right ventricular chamber are one third to one half of their counterpart in the left ventricle. Measurements can be obtained from long and short axis two-dimensional views and compared with normal values established in breeds of rabbits used as animal models for cardiovascular research (**Table 2**). The coronary sinus, which receives blood from the coronary veins and the left cranial vena cava, is very large and easily identified on the echocardiogram.[4] This apparently dilated coronary sinus, circling around the atrioventricular junction, should not be interpreted as a congenital defect or a sign of right-sided heart failure associated with elevated right atrial pressures. Blood flow within the heart and great vessels is assessed by Doppler echocardiography. Color flow Doppler, which

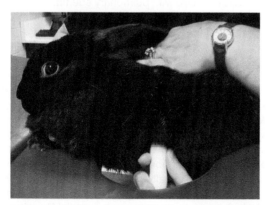

Fig. 2. Echocardiographic examination of the rabbit. The rabbit is gently restrained in sternal recumbency with the thorax positioned above a hole in the table. Echocardiographic examination is performed from beneath the animal.

Table 2
Values for echocardiographic variables in anesthetized rabbits with a mean weight of 2.59 kg[27]

Echocardiographic Variable	Mean (SD)
Interventricular septum diastole, mm	2.03 (0.37)
Interventricular septum systole, mm	3.05 (0.45)
Left ventricular free wall diastole, mm	2.16 (0.25)
Left ventricular free wall systole, mm	3.48 (0.45)
Left ventricular internal diameter diastole, mm	14.37 (1.49)
Left ventricular internal diameter systole, mm	10.05 (1.22)
Fractional shortening, %	30.13 (2.98)
Aortic diameter, mm	8.26 (0.76)
Left atrium, mm	9.66 (1.14)
Left atrium/aorta ratio	1.17 (0.14)

superimposes color-coded images of blood flow over two-dimensional images, facilitates the identification of regurgitant jets and shunts.

DISEASE PROCESSES AND TREATMENTS
Valvular Heart Disease

Chronic atrioventricular valve disease, also called endocardiosis, is more frequently identified in older rabbits. The mitral valve is the most commonly affected valve, but the lesions may also involve the tricuspid valve. Endocardiosis is defined as the thickening of the leaflets and lengthening of the chordae tendinae, which results in regurgitation of blood from the ventricle to the atrium during systole. On auscultation, a systolic murmur, usually heard best on the left sternal border, can be identified. The intensity of the murmur on auscultation may vary with the amount of regurgitant blood (louder if the valve insufficiency is more severe), the orientation of the regurgitant jet (an eccentric jet is louder than a centrally oriented jet), or the morphology of the patient (murmur intensity is decreased in obese rabbits). The natural history of the disease is unknown in the rabbit. It is likely that, similarly to dogs, the rate of progression is usually slow but variable between individuals, and some rabbits will progress to congestive heart failure with pulmonary edema. At the stage of congestive heart failure, the left atrium is severely dilated, and the contractility of the enlarged left ventricle is usually preserved.

Cardiomyopathies

Myocardial failure results from nutritional deficiencies; viral, bacterial, and protozoal infections; toxins; or stress.[10] Cardiomyopathies are classified as dilated, hypertrophic, or restrictive based on the appearance of the ventricles on echocardiogram or at necropsy.[8,10] Most forms of cardiomyopathy are observed in large breeding colonies of rabbits, or induced experimentally in rabbits used as models for research. Cardiomyopathy rarely causes cardiovascular disease in pet rabbits. In rabbits, cardiomyopathies are sporadically diagnosed, and a causative agent is rarely identified. Diagnosis of cardiomyopathy is usually made by echocardiography in rabbits that present with signs of left- or right-sided congestive heart failure, arrhythmias, and collapsing episodes. Alpha2-agonists may cause myocardial fibrosis and necrosis in the rabbit, but most studies don't confirm this suspicion.[13,14] The rabbit is very sensitive to stress and sudden death is sporadically reported by veterinarians. Some of these deaths may be a result of stress-induced cardiomyopathy. The effects of norepineph-rine on cardiac function have been extensively studied in the rabbit.[15] High levels of catecholamines cause coronary vasoconstriction and myocardial ischemia in the rabbit. To limit stress, the rabbit should always be kept in a quiet environment and han-dled in a gentle manner while in the hospital.

Arrhythmias

Arrhythmias may be associated with structural cardiac diseases. However, arrhyth-mias requiring treatment are uncommon in rabbits and only arrhythmias associated with clinical signs should be treated with antiarrhythmic drugs. Severe bradycardia or short bursts of rapid ventricular tachycardia may result in episodic weakness or syncope. Sustained tachycardia may cause myocardial failure over a few weeks. This has been demonstrated experimentally by rapid pacing of the right atrium or ven-tricle.[16] Chronic rapid pacing at rates between 350 and 400 beats/min over a period of several weeks produces myocardial depression and clinical signs of heart failure.[17] Severe bradycardia during anesthesia should be treated with glycopyrrolate, which may be more effective than atropine, as some rabbits produce atropinesterase, an en-zyme responsible for rapid hydrolysis of atropine.[18] High-grade atrioventricular block, characterized by many nonconducting P waves and pauses of a few seconds, may re-spond to oral theophylline or require pacemaker implantation if clinical signs of ex-ercise intolerance or syncope persist. Sustained supraventricular tachycardia, characterized by normal morphology QRS complexes with or without visible P waves, should be treated to slow the atrioventricular node conduction time and interrupt the travel of some of the rapid atrial impulses from atrium to ventricle. While digoxin is in-dicated, the possibility of toxicity necessitates measuring blood levels after a few days of treatment, 6 to 8 hours after the last dose. Alternatively, the rabbit can be watched for anorexia or gastrointestinal signs and the dose of digoxin decreased, or the med-ication stopped if those signs occur. Diltiazem is a calcium channel blocker also used to slow atrioventricular conduction and therefore heart rate. However, diltiazem de-creases myocardial contractility and may cause hypotension. Rapid ventricular tachy-cardia may respond to intravenous boluses of lidocaine. Mexiletine and sotalol, antiarrhythmics used in the management of canine ventricular arrhythmias, have been tested experimentally in rabbits, but their chronic use has not been evaluated in the pet rabbit.[19]

Congestive Heart Failure

As a prey species, the rabbit shows few overt signs of disease.[20] Therefore heart fail-ure is usually recognized at an advanced stage when the clinical signs become visible to the owner. Most rabbits with dyspnea have primary respiratory disease, most likely pasteurellosis, but congestive heart failure should be considered if respiratory signs are not associated with purulent ocular or nasal discharge. Open-mouthed breathing occurs only in significantly compromised animals, as rabbits are obligate nose breathers. Coughing is not a common presenting complaint in rabbits with severe car-diac enlargement.[8] Left-sided heart failure leads to pulmonary edema and dyspnea. Right-sided heart failure results in systemic venous congestion, which causes a distention of the veins on the ventral abdomen, and rarely exophtalmos secondary to the engorgement of the venous sinuses behind the eyes.[8] Pleural effusion is also a sign of right-sided failure.

Management of congestive heart failure requires long-term administration of various drugs. Intravenous medications can be injected through a small-gauge intravenous catheter placed in the cephalic vein, an auricular vein, or the lateral saphenous vein.[21] Intramuscular injections are given in the paralumbar muscles. For oral medications, it is preferable to use liquid formulations. Compounding pharmacies prepare customized medications. Bunny-favorite flavorings can be added to the solutions. To administer the medication, the rabbit should be restrained in a towel, its head elevated, and the medication should be injected with a syringe placed into the interdental space (diastema).[21] There are no cardiac drugs approved by the Food and Drug Administration (FDA) for use in rabbits. Moreover, the recommended dosages of most drugs are only based on the author's personal experience and extrapolation from canine and feline cardiology literature. Most cardiac medications used in dogs have been safely used in rabbits at similar dosages (**Table 3**). No medication has demonstrated a beneficial effect before the onset of congestive heart failure. Congestive heart failure is primarily managed with furosemide, a loop diuretic. It is administered intravenously in situations of acute pulmonary edema in addition to oxygen therapy. For long-term therapy, an angiotensin-converting enzyme (ACE) inhibitor is usually added to furosemide. ACE inhibitors counteract the activation of the renin angiotensin aldosterone system. A positive inotrope should be added to the treatment regimen if ventricular contractility is severely impaired. Pimobendan is a potent positive inotropic agent with vasodilatory properties. In the dog, pimobendan increases cardiac output and mesenteric and renal blood flow, and decreases diastolic ventricular pressures at a dose of 0.1 to 0.3 mg/kg.[22] Renal function should be monitored in patients treated with furosemide and an ACE inhibitor. The dose of furosemide must be adapted to the clinical response. It is always preferable to increase the frequency of furosemide administration rather than the dosage. Taurine supplementation at a dose of 100 mg/kg/day by mouth has been showed to markedly improve cardiac function in rabbits with artificially induced aortic regurgitation and secondary heart failure.[23] Therefore, some rabbits with spontaneous cardiac disease may benefit from daily administration of taurine.

Table 3
Recommended cardiovascular drugs for use in the rabbit

Drug	Approximate Dosage	Category	Major Indications	Comments
Furosemide	1–3 mg/kg q8–24h PO 1–4 mg/kg SC, IM, IV PRN	Loop diuretic	Congestive heart failure	Risk of hyponatremia, hypochloremia, hypokalemia
Enalapril	0.5 mg/kg q12–24h PO	ACE inhibitor	Congestive heart failure, hypertension	Monitor renal function
Digoxin	0.005 mg/kg q 12–24h PO	Positive inotrope, vagomimetic	Myocardial failure, supraventricular tachycardia	Monitor serum levels
Pimobendan	0.1–0.3 mg/kg q 12–24h PO	Positive inotrope, afterload reducer	Myocardial failure, congestive heart failure	
Diltiazem	0.5–1 mg/kg q 8–24h PO	Calcium channel blocker	Supraventricular tachycardia	Risk of bradycardia and hypotension
Lidocaine	1–2 mg/kg IV PRN	Sodium channel blocker	Ventricular tachycardia	Serum potassium must be normal

Abbreviations: IM, intramuscular; IV, intravenous; PO, orally; PRN, as needed; q, every; SC, subcutaneous.

Systemic Hypertension

Systemic hypertension is rarely reported but may occur in association with renal failure. It is usually controlled with an ACE inhibitor. Enalapril has been used in rabbits without major side effects. Anecdotal reports indicate a high sensitivity of the rabbit to the effects of benazepril.[8] Studies evaluating the safety of benazepril and its antiproliferative and antiatherogenic effects in rabbit models have used oral dosages of 1 mg/kg/day without major side effects.[24–26] However, the clinician should proceed with information cautiously, as laboratory animals may not have been evaluated clinically for activity level, or appetite.

SUMMARY

This article reviews what is known about the diagnosis and management of cardiovascular diseases in the pet rabbit. Current knowledge is based on anecdotal reports, derived from research data using the rabbit as an animal model of human cardiovascular diseases, but most importantly canine and feline cardiology. It is likely that, as cardiovascular diseases are more often recognized, more specific information will soon become available for the treatment of the pet rabbit with cardiac disease.

REFERENCES

1. Finking G, Hanke H. Nikolaj Nikolajewitsch Anitschkow (1885–1964) established the cholesterol-fed rabbit as a model for atherosclerosis research. Atherosclerosis 1997;135:1–7.
2. Hew KW, Keller KA. Postnatal anatomical and functional development of the heart: a species comparison. Birth Defects Res B 2003;68:309–20.
3. Simons RS. Lung morphology of cursorial and non-cursorial mammals: lagomorphs as a case study for a pneumatic stabilization hypothesis. J Morphol 1996;230:299–316.
4. James TN. Anatomy of the cardiac conduction system in the rabbit. Circ Res 1967;20:638–48.
5. Evans HE. The heart and arteries. In: Evans HE, editor. Miller's anatomy of the dog. 3rd edition. Philadelphia: WB Saunders; 1993. p. 586–681.
6. Manning PJ, Ringler DH, Newcomer CE. Cardiovascular system. In: Ringler DH, Manning PJ, Newcomer CE, editors. The biology of the laboratory rabbit. 2nd edition. San Diego (CA): Academic Press; 1994. p. 63.
7. Marano G, Grigioni M, Tiburzi F, et al. Effects of isoflurane on cardiovascular system and sympathovagal balance in New Zealand white rabbits. J Cardiovasc Pharmacol 1996;28:513–8.
8. Reusch B. Investigation and management of cardiovascular disease in rabbits. In Pract 2005;27:418–25.
9. Hyllier EV, Quesenberry KE. Basic anatomy, physiology and husbandry. In: Quesenberry K, Carpenter JW, editors. Ferrets, rabbits, and rodents. Clinical medicine and surgery. Philadelphia: WB Saunders; 1997. p. 147–67.
10. Orcutt CJ. Cardiovascular disorders. In: Meredith A, Flecknell P, editors. BSAVA manual of rabbit medicine and surgery. Gloucester (UK): BSAVA; 2006. p. 96–102.
11. Kittleson MD. Signalment, history, and physical examination. In: Kittleson MD, Kienle RD, editors. Small animal cardiovascular medicine. St. Louis (MO): Mosby; 1998. p. 36–46.
12. Sato k, Chatani F, Sato S. Circadian and short-term variabilities in blood pressure and heart rate measured by telemetry. J Auton Nerv Syst 1995;54:235–46.

13. Marini RP, Li X, Harpster NK, et al. Cardiovascular pathology possibly associated with ketamine/xylazine anesthesia in Dutch belted rabbits. Lab Anim Sci 1999;49: 153–60.
14. Orr HE, Roughan JV, Flecknell PA. Assessment of ketamine and medetomidine anaesthesia in the domestic rabbit. Vet Anaesth Analg 2005;32(5):271–9.
15. Jiang JP, Chen V, Downing SE. Modulation of catecholamine cardiomyopathy by allopurinol. Am Heart J 1991;122:115–21.
16. Liang CS, Mao W, Iwai C, et al. Cardiac sympathetic neuroprotective effect of desipramine in tachycardia-induced cardiomyopathy. Am J Physiol Heart Circ Physiol 2006;290:H995–1003.
17. Hasenfuss G. Animal models of human cardiovascular disease, heart failure and hypertrophy. Cardiovasc res 1998;39:60–76.
18. Harrison PK, Tattersall JE, Gosden E. The presence of atropinesterase activity in animal plasma. Naunyn Schmiedebergs Arch Pharmacol 2006;373:230–6.
19. Niwano S, Inuo K, Morohoshi Y, et al. Mexiletine protects myocardium during acute ischemia by opening sarcolemmal K-ATP channel: studies in closed-chest acute ischemia model in rabbits. J cardiovasc Pharmacol 2004;44:639–44.
20. Grint NJ, Murison PJ. A comparison of ketamine-midazolam and ketamine-medetomidine combinations for induction of anaesthesia in rabbits. Vet Anaesth Analg 2008;35:113–21.
21. Brown S. Clinical techniques in rabbits. Seminars in Avian and Exotic Pet Medicine 1997;6:86–95.
22. Van Meel JC, Diederen W. Hemodynamic profile of the cardiotonic agent pimobendan. J Cardiovasc Pharmacol 1989;14:S1–6.
23. Takihara K, Azuma J, Awata N, et al. Beneficial effect of taurine in rabbits with chronic congestive heart failure. Am Heart J 1986;112(6):1278–84.
24. Li J, Hirose N, Kawamura M, et al. Antiatherogenic effect of angiotensin converting enzyme inhibitor (benazepril) and angiotensin II receptor antagonist (valsartan) in the cholesterol-fed rabbits. Atherosclerosis 1999;143:315–26.
25. Li J, Wnachun C. Benazepril on tissue angiotensin-converting enzyme and cellular proliferation in restenosis after experimental angioplasty. J Cardiovasc Pharmacol 1997;30:790–7.
26. Yamamoto S, Takemori E, Hasegawa Y, et al. General pharmacology of the novel angiotensin converting enzyme inhibitor benazepril hydrochloride. Effects on cardiovascular, visceral and renal functions and on hemodynamics. Arzneimittelforschung 1991;41:913–23.
27. Fontes-Sousa APN, Bras-Silva C, Moura C, et al. M-mode and Doppler echocardiographic reference values for male New Zealand white rabbits. Am J Vet Res 2006;67(10):1725–9.

Index

Note: Page numbers of article titles are in **boldface** type.

Vet Clin Exot Anim 12 (2009) 145–169
doi:10.1016/S1094-9194(08)00072-8
1094-9194/08/$ – see front matter © 2009 Elsevier Inc. All rights reserved.

Moving?

Make sure your subscription moves with you!

To notify us of your new address, find your **Clinics Account Number** (located on your mailing label above your name), and contact customer service at:

E-mail: elspcs@elsevier.com

800-654-2452 (subscribers in the U.S. & Canada)
314-453-7041 (subscribers outside of the U.S. & Canada)

Fax number: 314-523-5170

Elsevier Periodicals Customer Service
11830 Westline Industrial Drive
St. Louis, MO 63146

*To ensure uninterrupted delivery of your subscription, please notify us at least 4 weeks in advance of move.

Our issues help you manage *yours.*

Every year brings you new clinical challenges.

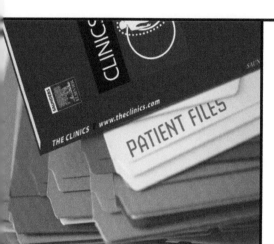

Every **Clinics** issue brings you **today's best thinking** on the challenges you face.

Whether you purchase these issues individually, or order an annual subscription (which includes searchable access to past issues online), the **Clinics** offer you an efficient way to update your know how…one issue at a time.

DISCOVER THE CLINICS IN YOUR SPECIALTY!

Veterinary Clinics of North America: Equine Practice.
Publishes three times a year.
ISSN 0749-0739.

Veterinary Clinics of North America: Exotic Animal Practice.
Publishes three times a year.
ISSN 1094-9194.

Veterinary Clinics of North America: Food Animal Practice.
Publishes three times a year.
ISSN 0749-0720.

Veterinary Clinics of North America: Small Animal Practice.
Publishes bimonthly.
ISSN 0195-5616.

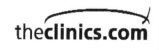